BREAKING
THE
FAT BARRIER

By Gordon S. Tessler, Ph.D.

DEDICATION

To the One True God and Father of us all, Who graciously gives us of His life and brings forth nutritious food from His earth.

To my precious wife, Laura, without whose love, prayers, and support, this book would not have been written. During the time this book was under construction she kept our home, cared for our three children, and still found the time to "trim the fat" out of this book.

ACKNOWLEDGMENTS

My heartfelt appreciation to Joe and Sara Call, Sandra Levinson, and Cal Mason for their willing sacrifice in service to the Lord and His desire to heal and restore His people.

A special thanks to Jennifer Philbeck, Blanca Richmond-Coca, and Beverly Mason for their research assistance. I am also grateful to Marsha Burt for her editing assistance. To all the clients of the Genesis Way, thank you for the many success stories that inspired me to write, **Breaking the Fat Barrier.**

TABLE OF CONTENTS

INTRODUCTION

"I'm allergic to food.
Every time I eat my skin breaks out in fat."
Jennifer Greene Duncan

Dieting has become the **Great American Obsession**. A national health survey recently reported that half the women and a quarter of the men in the United States are on some sort of diet.[1] One would expect from our preoccupation with getting those extra pounds off, that America would be populated with skinny people. Not so! Despite our dieting efforts, experts estimate that **two out of five people in the United States are overweight.** The diet industry reported earnings in excess of thirty billion dollars last year and why not. It is a business where you are practically guaranteed repeat customers!

For those who are a part of the "Diet Generation", "dieting" means "starvation" and starvation never works for very long! Art Buchwald, a well-known columnist, wrote that the word **"diet"** comes from the verb **"to die"**! Anyone who decides to "go on a diet" must realize that calories will have to be restricted, enjoyment for food will have to cease and hunger will be a constant friend. Who would want to live under those conditions?

Although it is obvious that calorie-restricted diets only work for the short term, we persist in trying another diet and another, expecting a different result. Even if we reach our weight goal, statistics tell us that 95 out of l00 people will put it all back on again! **In reality, we never lost the weight, we only misplaced it for a little while.**

Americans don't need another diet. We need to improve the one we have! Wholesome food choices have been replaced with pre-packaged foods which are laden with fat and sugar. The American Cancer Society and the American Heart Association believe that sixty to seventy percent of cancer and heart disease is diet-related. Positive food choices can reduce our risk of these and other degenerative diseases. **We need to turn our "deathstyle" of** living into a "lifestyle" that can reduce not only our weight, but also our risk of heart disease, strokes, cancer, and diabetes.[2]

The simple truth is that **diets don't work** and once we understand why, then we can find out what does. Dieters have put their faith in theories of weight loss which are simply not true. These myths of dieting have been sold to us even though recent research contradicts them. Numerous studies from research centers across America confirm that more calories, not less, are needed in order to improve your metabolism and ability to burn fat. Old myths die hard but **a new era is on the horizon for those who are truly ready for the common sense approach to safe, permanent fat loss and weight control.**

The Genesis Way is not a diet, it's a way of life! The word "genesis" means "beginning" and this will be a **"new beginning"** for you. This new lifestyle offers you a healthy, safe and permanent way to reduce excess bodyfat without dieting - turning your body into an efficient fat-burning furnace - **Breaking the Fat Barrier** once and for all!

Be well,

Gordon S. Tessler

CHAPTER ONE

WHY DIETING WON'T BREAK THE FAT BARRIER

*"I gained and lost the same ten pounds so many times...
my cellulite must have deja vu."*
James Wagner

Today Americans are eating fewer calories than eighty years ago, nevertheless, we are still gaining weight.[1] In the early 1980's, the Metropolitan Life Insurance Company increased the acceptable average weight three to twelve pounds for men and two to nine pounds for women on their height/weight charts. Clearly, the Gross National Product is not the only indicator of our nation's "growth"! Forty percent (40%) of all Americans are overweight and for most of them, dieting has become a way of life! Skipping meals and restricting calories is thought to be the only way to get rid of those extra pounds.

The Energy Balance Theory of Weight Loss

Cutting calories in order to lose weight is based on an old theory called the Energy Balance Theory. This traditional explanation of weight gain or loss is simple. The body is a passive container that takes in a certain number of calories each day and then uses them up through various activities.

According to this theory, if a person

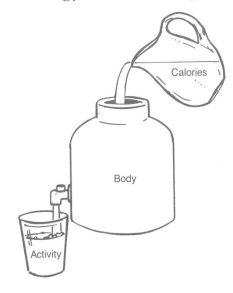

Energy Balance Theory

Calories

Body

Activity

takes in more calories than he burns, he gains weight. On the other hand, taking in fewer calories than needed results in lost weight. There are only two ways to lose weight based on the Energy Balance Theory: 1) decrease calories, while maintaining activity level or 2) increase activity level to burn more calories. This concept seems so logical that few have ever challenged it and yet, discoveries in food science and nutrition over the last twenty-five (25) years reveal significant fallacies in this theory of weight loss and gain. If the Energy Balance Theory were true then overweight people would eat more calories and exercise less than normal weight people. Nationwide studies find no relationship between overweight people and overeating.[2-4] According to one such study, the HANES I National Health and Nutrition Examination Survey, neither greater caloric intake nor decreased activity are causes of weight gain.[4]

When the Energy Balance Theory was first presented, people thought all calories were the same - a fat calorie was the same as a carbohydrate calorie was the same as a protein calorie. However, **all calories are not created equal!** For example, a gram of fat has 2.3 times as many calories as a gram of carbohydrate or protein. Our bodies are not passive containers as this theory suggests, but living organisms that process these different calories in different ways! The body stores certain calories in the fat and others in the muscle. Some calories burn quickly in the body while others burn for many hours. **Contrary to the Energy Balance Theory, the critical factor in permanent weight control is not the number of calories consumed but the composition of these calories.**

Calorie Restriction Unnecessary
While the dieting industry focuses on restricting all calories, scientific evidence suggests that fat calories are the real culprit in weight gain. Research has shown that changing the composition of the calories in our diet alters the body's ability to gain or lose weight.[5-12] **Since fat calories are the real culprit in gaining weight, limiting all calories, as most diet programs suggest, is totally unnecessary.** In fact, eating more, not less, of the right type of calories is absolutely necessary to boost one's metabolism in order to break the fat barrier.

Calorie Restriction Dangerous

When low-calorie diets are imposed, the body cannot distinguish between starvation and dieting.[13-17] It responds to dieting by conserving energy (slowing metabolism) and holding onto fat reserves. The body actually begins to "eat itself" (breaking down living tissue) because the calories in the diet do not provide enough energy. **Diets don't work because starvation is against the basic instinct to live!** No wonder so many people can't "stay" on a diet program. Their bodies will not let them starve to death!

Yo-Yo Dieting: Easier to gain, harder to lose!

In my many years as a clinical nutritionist, hundreds of women have complained to me that with each new diet they tried, it became harder to lose weight and much easier to regain it. The results of a study conducted in 1986 confirm what my clients have told me.[18] This study examined the effects of repeated dieting on obese female rats. These overweight rats were put on a calorie-restricted diet until they lost their extra weight, then they were allowed to resume their regular eating patterns. During the first round of dieting, the rats lost their excess weight in 21 days. After normal eating resumed, they gained it all back in 45 days. In the second round of dieting, the rats took 46 days to lose the same amount of weight and only 14 days to gain it all back! These results are consistent with the dieting dilemma that many chronic dieters experience.[19-20]

Yo-Yo Dieting Can Lead to Health Problems

The health risks associated with yo-yo dieting and weight fluctuation may now be more serious than those associated with excess weight. In a health study conducted over a 30 year period,[21] researchers came to some alarming conclusions: **those people whose body weight fluctuated greatly, or often, had a higher risk of coronary heart disease and death than those people with relatively stable body weight.** Any number of diets can take weight off but few are able to keep it off. The issue is not only weight loss, it's weight control!

Dieting Can Make You Fatter!

Not only is it more difficult to lose weight after the second, third, or fourth try, but these cycles of weight loss and weight gain can cause

diet-induced obesity. Obesity means more than just being overweight. It actually refers to excess bodyfat. A male whose bodyfat exceeds twenty percent (20%) and a female whose bodyfat exceeds twenty-five percent (25%) is considered "obese". It appears that repeated dieting makes the body more efficient at fat utilization and storage.[19, 20, 22] While dieting, the body tends to conserve fat and burn (or lose) lean muscle. When regular eating resumes, the body will regain the lost weight not as lean muscle but as fat! **The phenomenon of "yo-yo dieting" can actually make a person fatter!**

Americans are overfat, not just overweight!
The real problem is not in how much we weigh, but in how much excess bodyfat we have. A professional football player, who has "beefed up" his body by weight training, can be overweight. That extra weight can be healthy if it is rippling muscles or it can be unhealthy if it shows itself as double chins, thunder thighs, or potbellies. Fashion models, the ideal women to many Americans, are good examples of what calorie-restricted diets can do to your body. They are forever "dieting" to fit into those size eight designer clothes. Yet body composition tests on these models reveal a high percentage of bodyfat in relation to lean muscle. Their dieting efforts are "eating up" the lean muscle, not just the fat! **Therefore, losing weight does not necessarily mean you are losing unwanted fat pounds.**

Composition of Body Weight
Our body weight is composed of three parts: Muscle, Bone, and Fat. Do you know how many pounds of your total weight are muscle? How many are fat? Your bathroom scale cannot give you that kind of information.

COMPOSITION OF MUSCLE AND FAT[23]

	Water	Lipids (fats)	Protein
Muscle	70%	7%	22%
Fat	22%	72%	6%

Only muscle and fat can be changed to reflect a true weight loss or gain on your scale.   Muscle weighs 2.5 times more than fat because it consists mostly of water. Unfortunately, a significant amount of the weight lost while dieting is muscle and water - not fat! **Muscle is not the right kind of weight to lose since it is the most metabolically active tissue in your body!** Each muscle is like a little furnace, and the more lean muscle you have, the more efficient your body's ability to burn calories. **We must lose excess bodyfat, not muscle!**

In order to break the fat barrier, we must improve the composition of our weight by reducing the amount of excess bodyfat while increasing the amount of lean muscle. The Genesis Way provides a safe, healthy and permanent way to improve your body composition and avoid the weight cycling health hazards of calorie-restricted diet programs. **You can lose the "right" weight, the Genesis Way!**

CHAPTER TWO

COMMON MYTHS ABOUT DIETING

"You never know how much you really believe anything until its truth
or falsehood becomes a matter of life and death to you."
C.S. Lewis

Myth #1   **Eating too many calories causes you to become
overweight.**

Actually, the number of calories you eat is not the cause of obesity.
To counter the U. S. trend toward obesity, the U.S. Department of
Agriculture and the U.S. Department of Health and Human
Services, in a publication entitled NUTRITION AND YOUR HEALTH
- DIETARY GUIDELINES FOR AMERICANS, recommend reducing
the fat content of our diets, not the total calories.[1-2] Cross-cultural
studies show that obesity is more widespread in societies that
consume a greater proportion of calories from dietary fat.[3-4] Forty-
two percent (42%) of all calories in the American diet come from
dietary fat! In China, where there is little obesity, the Chinese
consume twenty percent (20%) more calories than Americans but
only fifteen percent (15%) of those calories come from dietary fat.

Myth #2   **The overweight and the obese are fat because they
eat more and exercise less.**

Between 1971 and 1975, the HANES I Survey evaluated the caloric
intake, activity level and body weight of several thousand American
citizens (20,749)[5]. This nutritional study found a clear relationship
between body weight and caloric intake, but not the one you would
expect! Thin people in the survey ate many more calories than the
overweight subjects. In fact, the more obese the people were, the
fewer calories they ate! Many studies demonstrate that overweight
people eat less, or certainly no more, calories than nonobese
people. [5-9] **Investigators in all these scientific studies do not
support the common belief that gluttony and laziness cause
obesity.**

Myth #3   Cutting calories leads to loss of bodyfat.

Dieting can actually make you fatter! Your basal metabolic rate, or BMR, is the number of calories you need per day to maintain your basic body functions when you are at rest. Most experts agree that women need at least 1000 calories per day and men need a minimum of 1200 calories per day to maintain BMR. Because men have more muscle mass than women, their metabolisms require more calories. To compute your own BMR is quite simple. Adult men require eleven calories each day for every pound of body weight and women require ten calories per pound to maintain their BMR. For example, a woman that weighs 120 pounds needs 1200 calories to maintain life's essential body functions. Of course, that's if she doesn't move! But if she does anything more than just lie still, more calories are needed above and beyond her BMR.

Most weight loss programs give their participants calorie restricted regimes of between 500 to 1000 calories a day. We don't have to be rocket scientists to figure out that a diet of 500, 800, or 1000 calories a day will not support the basic body functions.   Reducing caloric intake causes the body to conserve calories in order to maintain basic body functions, thereby slowing the metabolism. The body slows its metabolism, holds onto fat reserves, and uses the protein and sugar in the muscles. A recent study at the Vanderbilt University School of Medicine found that chronic dieters had less muscle mass and lower metabolic rates, while they often carried extra bodyfat around the waist area.[10] **A significant amount of the weight lost on calorie-restricted diets is not fat, but lean muscle and water**. After periods of fasting or caloric restriction, the body prefers to increase the fat enzyme, lipase, and add more pounds of fat instead of rebuilding the lost muscle.[11-14] Weight cycling (yo-yo dieting) studies have found that repeating calorie-restricted diets "may lead to permanent metabolic changes which promote weight gain (fat gain) and make subsequent loss of weight more difficult". [15-17]

8

Myth #4   Exercise helps you lose weight.

Actually exercise can make you heavier since exercising builds muscle. Muscle weighs 2.5 times more than fat. The added muscle may show up on your bathroom scale as extra weight. But take heart! You will replace excess bodyfat with lean muscle. A lean body makes you look and feel better! You will also lose inches around the waist, thighs and hips. Dress sizes will go down as well as pants and suit sizes. With those kind of results, who cares how much weight you have lost!

Myth #5   Combining exercise with a low-calorie diet is the perfect marriage that guarantees weight loss.

Low-calorie diets are low energy diets! Who feels like exercising on a starvation diet? If you did not feel like exercising before dieting, what makes you think you will feel like exercising while eating a diet that does not even support the basic bodily functions? On a calorie-deficient diet the body wants to conserve energy, not increase its activity by exercising more!

Myth #6   Your dieting efforts failed because you did not have enough will power and self control.

Suppose someone told you that you could lose ten pounds if you could just hold your breath for ten minutes? Sound crazy? The basic survival instinct of your body would force you to start breathing again. If they accused you of not having enough will power, you would know that was ridiculous! Similarly, a commercial promises that you can lose all your excess weight by going on their low-calorie diet program. So, you pay the fee, start the diet, and after a few days or weeks, you go off the diet. Your body needed more calories than the diet provided. It was not that you needed more self-control or will power, you just could not exist for very long on a starvation diet. **Diets don't work because starvation is against the basic instinct to live!**

Myth #7   Carbohydrates are fattening!

On the contrary! Even after a 2,000 calorie carbohydrate meal, less than one percent (1%) was converted into fat.[20-21] It takes four times the amount of energy for the body to store carbohydrates as fat than it does to convert them into glucose for fuel.[9, 18, 19] Obesity is very rare in geographical areas where high complex carbohydrate diets are eaten. Research data concludes that eating a high carbohydrate diet does not lead to obesity in humans.[20-25]

Myth #8   Height/Weight charts tell you how much you should weigh.

The problem with these charts is that they ignore body composition! Just because you fall in the correct range for your height and weight does not mean that you have the correct balance of bodyfat to muscle. The ratio of bodyfat to lean muscle is far more important to your health than simply how much you weigh. Your correct weight is determined by the average percent of bodyfat for your age. Since muscle weighs 2.5 times more than fat, a person could be "overweight" if he has too much muscle. Too much muscle is not a health risk; too much bodyfat is!

Myth #9   All calories are the same. A calorie is a calorie is a calorie!

A few years ago scientists and nutritionists believed that all calories were created equal, regardless of their source. Studies now prove that calories are handled differently in the body.[20-26] Dietary fat has twice as many calories as carbohydrates. The body prefers to convert the dietary fat into bodyfat and the carbohydrates into muscle.

Conclusion

As newer and more accurate scientific research corrects misunderstandings and myths about dieting, we are left with the question, "What is the truth about weight gain and weight loss?" To answer such an important question we must begin with an understanding of metabolism and its relationship to the overweight person.

CHAPTER THREE

THERMOGENESIS: THE FIRE THAT BOOSTS YOUR METABOLISM

"I told my doctor I get tired when I go on a diet, so he gave me pep pills. Know what happened? I ate faster."
Joe E. Lewis

Metabolism plays a key role in the body's ability to lose weight. The Energy Balance Theory states that there are only two ways to lose weight - eat less or exercise more. However, the very act of eating changes your metabolism! Every time you eat, your body produces heat to burn calories.[1] This production of heat is called **thermogenesis.**[2] The majority of thermogenesis (up to 90%) takes place in the muscle.[3] Eating produces the fire of thermogenesis which boosts the metabolic rate in your body. **Food stimulates thermogenesis and thermogenesis stimulates your metabolism.**[4]

Reduced Thermogenesis in the Overweight
Many scientists and researchers from all over the world have found that **obesity is directly related to reduced thermogenesis.**[5-13] This means that the production of heat which is normally generated after a meal is too low. Because of reduced thermogenesis, the metabolism is slowed and less calories are burned. That is why overweight people have been insisting for years that they have a slower metabolism.

Fuel for Thermogenesis
There are two kinds of fuel or energy burned in the muscle during thermogenesis. One type of fuel is glucose (sugar), which comes from simple and complex carbohydrates. The other type of fuel is fat stored in the bodyfat.

Thermogenesis

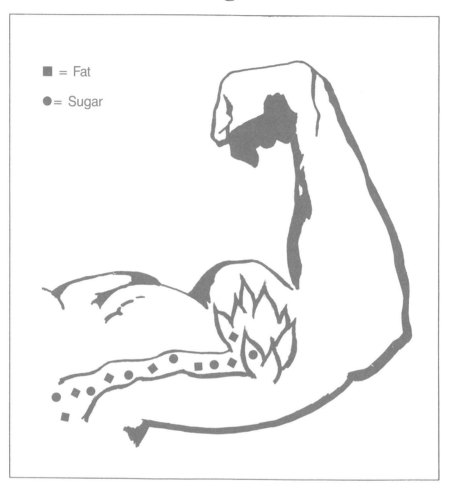

■ = Fat

● = Sugar

Insulin Important in Thermogenesis

The results of several studies also suggest that the hormone insulin plays an important role in thermogenesis.[14-22] Insulin helps the muscle cells receive both glucose and fat. After the muscle burns all the glucose, it begins to burn stored fat. In the overweight, for some unknown reason, insulin is not used properly to supply the muscles with adequate glucose and fat. This results in reduced thermogenesis. The overweight may have intense cravings for sugary foods because of the lack of sufficient fuel entering their cells. Starchy complex carbohydrates in the diet are the best type of food for the overweight since they lower the need for insulin [17, 18, 23-25] and reduce sweet cravings.

Factors to Boost Thermogenesis

1. Frequency of calories eaten

According to studies, every time you eat a snack or a meal, your metabolic rate goes up as the heat of thermogenesis fires up your metabolism![26-28] As you eat more calories, more often, you are putting your metabolism in **high gear!** Instead of decreasing calories which slows your metabolism, we need to stoke the fires of thermogenesis. **Stop starving and start stoking!** By eating more often the Genesis Way, you will fire up thermogenesis and boost your metabolism to burn more calories!

2. Type of Calories Eaten

Fat Calories

Of the 3 types of calories you can eat, fat is the major enemy of thermogenesis. Dietary fat has a much less thermogenic effect than either carbohydrates or protein.[22, 24, 29] Studies done on both animals and humans have shown that the higher the percentage of fat in the diet, the lower the thermogenic response to food.[11, 22, 24] In other words, **fat is not a good thermogenic food.** Too much dietary fat slows our metabolism!

Carbohydrate Calories

Carbohydrate calories are the preferred fuel to fire thermogenesis. Results from many studies demonstrate that our bodies are designed to accommodate large amounts of carbohydrates.[18, 23-25] The body burns carbohydrates as energy in the muscle rather than storing them as bodyfat. Of the three types of calories, **carbohydrates are the most thermogenic.**

Protein Calories

The proteins eaten in America come primarily from dairy products and red meats. Unfortunately, they are accompanied by a large percentage of fat! We have already learned that dietary fat does not contribute to increased thermogenesis; therefore, the best proteins for thermogenesis are ones that contain only small amounts of fat. The best choices for protein are beans, legumes, the whites of eggs, skinless chicken and turkey, and fin and scale fish. The beans and legumes have little fat content while the chicken, turkey and fish have about half the fat, or less, of most red meats.

Conclusion

In order to boost metabolism, thermogenesis must increase. In order to increase thermogenesis, adequate calories must be consumed. In fact, limiting calories can reduce thermogenesis. Carbohydrates are the best thermogenic foods to boost metabolism and are the least likely to be stored as fat. Therefore, they should be consumed frequently during the day. The composition of our diets should be primarily complex carbohydrates (65%-70%), a moderate amount of low-fat protein (l0%-l5%), and very little total fat (15%-20%). **The proper composition of our calories will insure a lean, healthy body with a "high performance" metabolism!**

CHAPTER FOUR

FORGET CALORIES, THINK FAT: THE REAL CAUSE OF OBESITY

"Fat is not a moral problem. It's an oral problem."
Jane Thomas Noland

While the total caloric intake of our diets has gone down, the percent of total calories from fat has gone up. Time-trend data for the United States show that the percent of fat in the American diet increased from thirty-two percent (32%) to forty-three percent (43%) between 1915 and 1985.[1-2] On a yearly basis, this increase is equal to twenty-four pounds of fat per person! Studies show that ninety-seven percent (97%) of all dietary fat is converted into bodyfat. Fat cells can expand ten to twenty times their normal size to accommodate these large amounts of fat. The reason that Americans are overweight is simple - **they eat too much fat!**

The determining factor in weight gain is not the total number of calories consumed, but rather the total number of fat calories consumed. High fat means high calorie. A gram of fat has 2.3 times more calories than either a gram of protein or a gram of carbohydrate.

1 gram of protein = 4 calories
1 gram of carbohydrate = 4 calories
1 gram of fat = 9 calories

Researchers have found that the overweight do not eat more calories than normal weight people; however, they do consume more high fat foods.[3] In a recent Harvard study, the results were simply stated: "we suggest that fat intake may play a role in obesity that is independent of total energy (or caloric) intake."[4] **Calories don't make you fat - fat makes you fat!**

Experimental research strongly supports the association between lowered dietary fat intake and weight loss. One such study, the

Women's Health Trial, examined the effects of long-term reduction of dietary fat on weight loss. None of the women who participated in this study were following a low-fat diet. Their average intake of dietary fat was thirty-nine percent (39%). One group of women reduced their total dietary fat to twenty percent (20%) and also increased their total intake of carbohydrates and protein. This group reduced fats in cooking and flavoring, substituted low or nonfat foods for high-fat foods, and increased the use of fish, chicken, grains, fruits and vegetables in their diets. The participants were reviewed at six months, one year, and two years. The group who continued their usual thirty-nine percent (39%) calories from fat, showed little change in weight. The women who substantially reduced their fat intake (from 39% to 20%), while increasing their carbohydrate intake, lost weight. "These results suggest that a low-fat diet (20%), which does not overly restrict caloric intake, may be a useful component in weight-loss regimens."[3] **Weight loss and weight control are directly related to a restriction in dietary fat and not a restriction in total calories.** The Genesis Way recommends that dietary fat compose fifteen to twenty percent (15% -20%) of the total calories eaten.

Fats: The Good, The Bad and The Ugly

Good Fats - Essential Fatty Acids
There are two types of fats used in the body: essential fatty acids (EFAs) and nonessential fatty acids. Nonessential fatty acids are manufactured by the body; essential fatty acids are not. There are only two essential fatty acids and they must come from your food! These two essential fatty acids are: Linoleic Acid (LA) and Linolenic Acid (LNA).

Linoleic Acid (LA)
Linoleic acid, commonly referred to as omega-6 fatty acid, is present in dairy products, organ meats, human milk, and most notably in vegetable seed oils such as sunflower, safflower, corn and soy oil. Olive oil, a rich source of omega-9 monosaturated fatty acids, contains a small amount of LA. Palm and coconut oil contain none![5] Insufficient amounts of LA in the diet can cause: eczema-like skin eruptions, loss of hair, liver and kidney degeneration,

excessive sweating accompanied by thirst, slow wound healing, susceptibility to infections, sterility in men and miscarriages in women, arthritis, heart and circulatory problems, and slow growth.

Linolenic Acid (LNA)

The popular name for linolenic acid is omega-3 fatty acid. Fish oils have the highest concentrations of omega-3 fatty acids. The Greenland Eskimos, whose diet consists primarily of fish, seal, and whale, have been the focus of much research in the last few years. Despite the fact that their diet is high in cholesterol and fat, these Eskimos have a very low incidence of coronary heart disease.[6] Omega-3 fish oils are one of the good fats for a healthy heart.

Linolenic acid is also found in human milk and the seed oil of the evening primrose as gamma-linolenic acid or GLA. Alpha-linolenic acid, or ALA, is present in a variety of grains and soy oil although food manufacturers hydrogenate it. The hydrogenation process leads to a loss of essential fatty acid activity.[5] Deficiencies of LNA can cause weakness, impaired vision, learning disabilities, motor incoordination, tingling in arms and legs, and behavioral changes.

Essential Fatty Acids-A Final Word

Sufficient amounts of fat are needed in the diet to provide the essential fatty acids that your body cannot manufacture.[6] Much is still unknown about the importance of EFAs in various body functions, but we do know that they are vital for good health. The following is a partial list of their benefits:

* Needed to assimilate certain fat soluble vitamins-A, D, E, F, and K
* Act like "magnets" to attract oxygen into the body
* Hold oxygen in the cell membranes deterring both viruses and bacteria
* Involved in all gland secretions including insulin and sex hormones
* Hold proteins in cell membranes
* Help carry nutrients in and out of the cells
* Required for metabolism of all normal tissue

Essential fatty acids increase the metabolism of the body when they compose at least twelve to fifteen percent (12%-15%) of the total calories. Every individual who desires to turn his body into a **fat-burning furnace** needs essential fatty acids for an efficient metabolism!

Bad Fats

The overconsumption of saturated fats, as in the Standard American Diet (S.A.D.), contributes to coronary heart disease, strokes, and cancer. Saturated fats are primarily found in animal products such as meats, dairy products, and eggs. All of these products are sources of cholesterol. Coconut and palm-kernel oils, found in many health food candies, are also sources of high saturated fats! These fats inhibit and block the activity of essential fatty acid functions in the body.[5,8]

Ugly Fats

Americans have significantly increased their consumption of polyunsaturated vegetable oils in an effort to cut both cholesterol and saturated fat from their diets. However, the overwhelming majority of these vegetable oils are in the form of **hardened vegetable fat!** Vegetable oil is naturally liquid at room temperature. So how do we get sticks of vegetable margarine? The process of **hydrogenation** forces hydrogen molecules into the structure of the polyunsaturated vegetable oil at 250 degrees or more! As a result, "new" fats or **trans-fats** are created. These trans-fatty acids are no longer polyunsaturated but now resemble saturated fatty acids.[9] The trans-fats help turn a liquid oil into a semi-solid or solid margarine. Hydrogenation allows a manufacturer to buy a cheap vegetable oil and **transform** it into a product that can compete with butter. Margarine, unlike butter, has a slightly rancid taste due to the high temperature hydrogenation process. These "man-made" trans-fats can actually contribute to cardiovascular disease and inhibit normal essential fatty acid metabolism.[9-16] The Genesis Way would rather you eat a pat of butter occasionally, instead of a "man-made" trans-fat like margarine.

Fat Facts

1.   High fat diets promote obesity.

Research shows that almost all dietary fat eaten goes immediately into fat storage.[19] The body only requires three percent (3%) of its energy to convert dietary fat in bodyfat. On the other hand, the body requires twenty-three percent (23%) of its energy to convert carbohydrates to fat storage. **Since carbohydrates are not easily converted into fat, they are the preferred calories!** Cross-cultural studies demonstrate that obesity is more common in societies that consume a greater proportion of their calories from dietary fat.[3] Changing the composition of the calories in the diet to more complex carbohydrates, with an emphasis on whole grains, will decrease the tendency to become overweight. **Remember, fat is fat and ninety-seven percent (97%) of fat calories are stored in the fat!**[20]

2.   High-fat diets produce low amounts of energy in comparison to high carbohydrate diets.

Research has shown that people on high carbohydrate diets can exercise three times longer than people on high fat diets.[21]

3.   It's your "fat tooth" that gets you in trouble, not your "sweet tooth"!

Most "sweet treats" are high in fat not just sugar! Fat, not sugar, provides the majority of calories in such sweet treats as ice cream, cookies, pastries, and candy. Sugar hides the unpleasant, oily taste of fat in a sweet, palatable form. How else could we swallow all that fat?

4.   Too much fat suppresses your metabolism.

The higher the percentage of fat in the diet, the lower the thermogenic response to food.[3,22] Eating too much fat will quench the fires of thermogenesis, thus slowing your metabolism.

5. Excess bodyfat increases your health risks.

Health organizations, such as the American Heart Association and the American Cancer Society, recommend lowering total dietary fat. Excess bodyfat contributes to increased risks of degenerative diseases such as heart disease, cancer, strokes, obesity, and diabetes.[2] This knowledge alone should motivate all of us to reduce the fat in our diets.

6. "Cholesterol Free", does not mean "Fat Free"!

Cholesterol-free products may contain the same amount of total fat as the cholesterol version. All foods that come from the seed of plants are cholesterol free. However, they still may contain vegetable fat.

Conclusion on Fats

The main point to remember when using any oil or fat is to use less of it. Ounce for ounce, pound for pound, fat is fat. Our bodies seem to be designed by our Creator to easily store dietary fat in the bodyfat! However, essential fatty acids from fish, like salmon, and non-hydrogenated vegetable oils, like safflower and olive oil, are needed for arterial health. Olive oil, used for thousands of years, has been helpful in lowering total cholesterol.[17] There is a need for adequate fat in the diet. The Surgeon General's Report on Nutrition and Health (1988) sums it up: "Adults need a minimum daily intake of fifteen to twenty-five grams of fat."[18] **Just remember the good fats for good health!**

Fatty Acid Composition of Oils and Fats
% of Total Fatty Acids

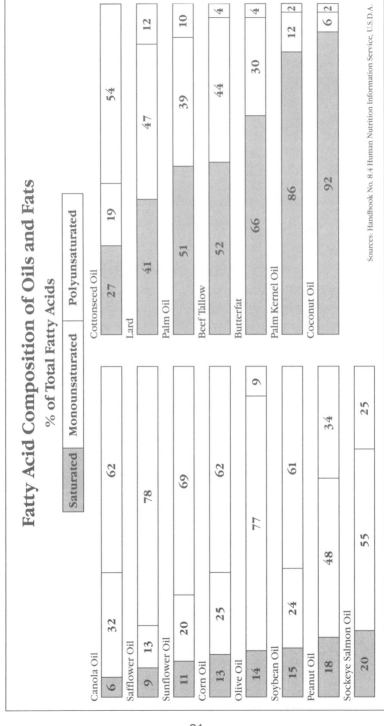

| Saturated | Monounsaturated | Polyunsaturated |

Canola Oil — 6 | 32 | 62

Safflower Oil — 9 | 13 | 78

Sunflower Oil — 11 | 20 | 69

Corn Oil — 13 | 25 | 62

Olive Oil — 14 | 77 | 9

Soybean Oil — 15 | 24 | 61

Peanut Oil — 18 | 48 | 34

Sockeye Salmon Oil — 20 | 55 | 25

Cottonseed Oil — 27 | 19 | 54

Lard — 41 | 47 | 12

Palm Oil — 51 | 39 | 10

Beef Tallow — 52 | 44 | 4

Butterfat — 66 | 30 | 4

Palm Kernel Oil — 86 | 12 | 2

Coconut Oil — 92 | 6 | 2

Sources: Handbook No. 8.4 Human Nutrition Information Service, U.S.D.A.

CHAPTER FIVE

PROTEIN: HOW MUCH IS ENOUGH?

A comment on the liquid diet fad:
"The powder is mixed with water and tastes exactly like powder
mixed with water."
Art Buchwald

Americans tend to eat far more protein than they need. For
instance, the "All American" breakfast might be two eggs, a three-
ounce slice of ham or bacon, a glass of milk, and two slices of toast,
totaling 42.3 grams of protein. The average adult needs
somewhere between 40-60 grams of protein a day. This breakfast
alone supplies adequate protein for an entire day! Lunch might be
a quarter-pound hamburger with a slice of cheese, totaling 29.8
grams of protein. Dinner might consist of an eight ounce T-bone
steak with a baked potato and broccoli. This dinner provides 61.1
grams of protein. Computing the protein content of these "three-
square" meals, we have a not-so-grand total of 133.2 grams of
protein. This hypothetical, but not unrealistic, menu contains three
times as much protein as the RDA requirement! Also, the 114.3
grams of fat contained in this menu represents more than twice the
amount of fat for men and more than three times the amount of fat
for women, that is recommended by the Genesis Way!

We need far less protein than we think. During a period of life when
protein is in great demand, nature supplies a surprisingly small
amount. Babies who triple their weight in the first year of life only
receive three to six percent protein from mother's milk, nature's
most perfect food for babies. By the time we reach nineteen years
of age, our protein requirement is only .8 grams per each 2.2
pounds of body weight. For example, a 110 pound woman needs
40 grams of protein per day, unless she is pregnant or lactating.
The danger is eating too much protein in the Standard American
Diet (S.A.D), not too little.

Risks from Overconsumption of Protein
Although protein deficiencies are almost unheard of in the United

States, protein excesses are commonplace. Consequently, there are certain risks associated with the overconsumption of protein.

1. Diets high in protein increase the body's loss of calcium. Excess phosphorous depletes calcium. The ideal ratio for the human body is 2 parts calcium to 1 part phosphorous. The ratio of calcium to phosphorous in meat is 1 part calcium to 20 parts phosphorous.
2. The higher a person's intake of meat and dairy products, the more grains, vegetables, and fruits will be crowded out of the diet. The lack of enough grains, vegetables, and fruits could cause possible vitamin and mineral deficiencies.
3. The human body has no adequate way to eliminate large quantities of excess protein. The liver and the kidneys must work harder to accommodate this overload.
4. Animal protein is accompanied by large amounts of fat. Too much fat in the diet has been associated with an increased risk of heart disease, cancer, strokes, and obesity. Although most people believe meat to be a protein food, further study reveals a surprising fact. A quarter-pound hamburger contains 28 grams of protein and 23 grams of fat. Because fat offers twice as many calories as protein, a hamburger contains 112 calories from protein and 207 calories from fat! Hamburgers are really "fat burgers." **Consumers of high meat and dairy diets tend to be overweight.**

Substitute Fish and Poultry
Poultry and fish provide high quality protein with a lower fat content than meat. The Genesis Way recommends reducing red meat consumption to one meal a month and eliminating pork altogether. By limiting fish (no shellfish) to three meals a week and poultry to four meals a week, we make room for more grains, vegetables, and fruits rich in fiber, vitamins and minerals.

Complete Vegetable Proteins
Beans and legumes are often referred to as "poor man's meat," but there is nothing poor about their protein quality. Beans, peas, and lentils are all fruits found within the pods of leguminous plants. Legumes, sometimes called pulses, have been eaten for thousands of years. They were cultivated in the Tigris-Euphrates Valley nearly four thousand years ago and are referred to in the Bible. Pureed

lentils or split peas are called "dal" in India. They are high in protein, and have been eaten regularly in the East Indian diet for thousands of years. Pureed chick-peas or garbanzo beans have been a staple in Arab and South American countries for centuries. Beans and legumes are all **fat-free** and can be substituted for any high protein meat.

Cooking Time for Beans and Legumes

Regular Bean	Pot Cooking Time	Pressure Cooking Time	Water	Amount Dry Beans	Yield
Black beans	1½ hours	20-25 min.	4 cups	1 cup	2 cups
Black-eyed peas	1 hour	20-25 min.	3 cups	1 cup	2 cups
Pinto beans	2½ hours	20-25 min.	3 cups	1 cup	2 cups
Kidney beans	1½ hours	20-25 min.	3 cups	1 cup	2 cups
Soybeans	3 hrs. or more	20-25 min.	3 cups	1 cup	2 cups
Garbanzo beans	3 hours	40-45 min.	4 cups	1 cup	4 cups
Lentils & Split peas	1 hour	10-15 min.	3 cups	1 cup	2¼ cups
Great Northern beans	2 hours	20-25 min.	3½ cups	1 cup	2 cups
Navy beans	1½ hours	20-25 min.	3 cups	1 cup	2 cups
Lima beans	1½ hours	20-25 min.	2 cups	1 cup	1¼ cups

*To make less musical, all beans and legumes should be soaked **at least** 12 hours. Pour off water, add water and cook. Cooking beans and legumes with a piece of kelp or other sea vegetable helps reduce musical quality also.

Eat Beans for Lowfat Protein

Beans and legumes play a vital role in the Genesis Way of life. Because of their high quality protein and very low fat content, they make an ideal substitute for animal protein. Also, the fact that they cost a fraction of what meat does, makes them affordable for everyone. Complex carbohydrates can be combined with beans or legumes for delicious and healthy meals.

CHAPTER SIX

CARBOHYDRATES: THE THERMOGENIC FUEL

"God said, See, I have given you **every plant** that **yields seed** which is on the face of all the earth, and **every tree** whose fruit **yields seed**, to you it shall be for food."
Genesis 1: 29

Human beings have lived primarily on grains, vegetables, and fruits for thousands of years. These unprocessed carbohydrates were created for the immediate and long-term energy requirements of our bodies. Without an abundance of carbohydrates, there would not be sufficient energy to live, work, or enjoy life. In fact, high carbohydrate diets provide three times the amount of energy as diets high in fat.[1] Unfortunately, over the past eighty years, carbohydrates, especially grains, have been pushed out of our diets in favor of fat.[2] These time-released energy foods are an important key to the Genesis Way of life. **In order to break the fat barrier, carbohydrates must regain their rightful place in our diets.**

There are two kinds of carbohydrates, simple and complex. The simple carbohydrates are like kindling to a fire. They get you going, but they don't last very long. Complex carbohydrates, on the other hand, are like logs in a fire. They burn slowly for a long time.

Simple Carbohydrates
The **simple carbohydrates** are short chains of sugar molecules called monosaccharides and disaccharides. Simple carbohydrates are nothing more than sugar in different forms (glucose, fructose, sucrose, and others). Fructose is a monosaccaride found in fruits and their juices. The most common disaccharides are refined sugar, honey, and molasses. Simple carbohydrates digest quickly and cause a greater and faster rise in glucose and insulin levels compared to the slower digesting complex carbohydrates.[3-4] In other words, simple carbohydrates take the express lane to the blood stream while complex carbohydrates must be broken down from starch into glucose.

CHANGES IN NUTRIENT CONSUMPTION
Per Capita for U.S. 1910-1976

CALORIES	1910-76	−3%
FAT	1910-76	+28%
CARBOHYDRATES	1910-76	−21%
PROTEIN	1910-76	+1%
DIETARY FAT from separated fats (butter, margarine, oil etc.)	1921-76	+56%
CARBOHYDRATES Grams (from sugars)	1909-13-1976	+31%
CARBOHYDRATES Grams (from starches)	1909-13-1976	−45%

Source: *Changing American Diet* by the Center for Science in the Public Interest.

Many people experience a burst of energy after a candy bar or other simple carbohydrates, only to feel an energy "crash" twenty minutes later. This "crash" is the body's way of lowering a high glucose level with insulin. **A diet high in simple carbohydrates puts a continual demand on insulin reserves**. Studies have

Simple Carbohydrates

Complex Carbohydrates

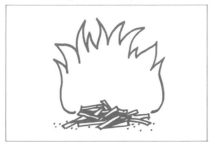

Short Burst of Energy

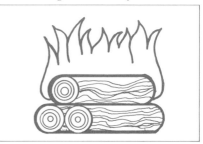

Long-lasting Energy

shown that the overweight have a problem with insulin reserves.[5-12] Perhaps the overconsumption of simple carbohydrates has caused this insulin sensitivity.

Simple carbohydrates give the body a "burst" of energy, but they cannot sustain that energy for very long. A quick sugar "fix" followed by a "low" leaves a person hungry for more simple sugars. **Thus, simple carbohydrates are not well suited for the overweight person.**

Simple Sugars Can Become Stored Fat

Just as dietary fat easily converts into bodyfat, so do simple carbohydrates! Simple carbohydrates enter the bloodstream very rapidly. The sudden flood of glucose requires a flood of insulin to handle it. The quicker insulin enters the bloodstream, the greater the likelihood that some of the simple carbohydrates will be stored as fat. The process of converting food into fat is called lipogenesis, which literally means "the birth of fat"! Too much fruit, fruit juices, high fructose corn syrup, fruit juice sweetened "healthy" treats, or refined sugar can be converted into fat and cause a weight gain. **The Genesis Way recommends that a person limit his simple carbohydrate intake to one fruit a day, preferably an apple, for the first ninety days.** At least whole fruit, unlike fruit juice, is rich in fiber which helps slow down the effects of the simple carbohydrates it contains. After the initial ninety day period, no more than two whole fruits a day are recommended.

Complex Carbohydrates

Complex carbohydrates are called polysaccharides. The body must break down these polysaccharides slowly because they are longer and more complex chains of sugar. The best complex carbohydrates are composed mostly of fiber and starch. The slow and gradual process of converting starch into glucose requires smaller amounts of insulin than the simple carbohydrates. Since studies confirm that overweight people have glucose and insulin difficulties, complex carbohydrates are more suited for them.[3] Whole fruits, vegetables, and starches are all complex carbohydrates. Starches include such foods as rice, barley, oats, potatoes, breads and pastas. Some starchy carbohydrates like potatoes, pasta, and bread create a greater rise in both glucose and

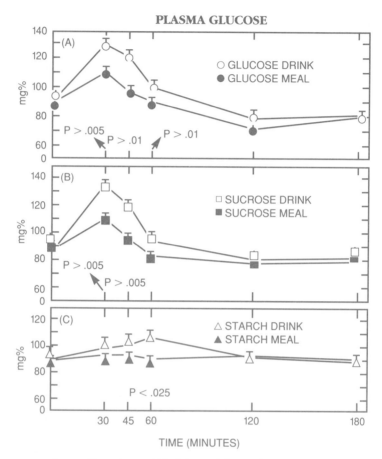

PLASMA GLUCOSE

Source: Department of Medicine and Clinical Research Center, Stanford University Medical Center, *Plasma Glucose and Insulin Responses to Orally Administered Simple and Complex Carbohydrates.*

insulin than do grains. Rice starch, for instance, has a much lower insulin and glucose response than potato starch.[3] Therefore, grains should be eaten in preference to other starchy carbohydrates in order to reduce bodyfat and control hunger.

Unprocessed Carbohydrates are not Fattening
For those who diet, carbohydrates are thought to be taboo foods. However, only the processed and refined carbohydrates are fattening because they contain so much added sugar and fat. For example, a potato is a good, starchy carbohydrate containing

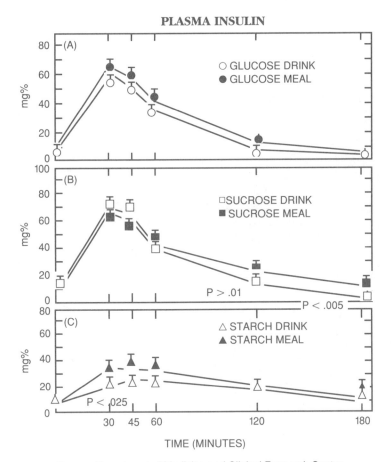

PLASMA INSULIN

(A)

○ GLUCOSE DRINK
● GLUCOSE MEAL

(B)

□ SUCROSE DRINK
■ SUCROSE MEAL

$P > .01$

$P < .005$

(C)

△ STARCH DRINK
▲ STARCH MEAL

$P < .025$

30 45 60   120   180

TIME (MINUTES)

Source: Department of Medicine and Clinical Research Center,
Stanford University Medical Center, *Plasma Glucose and Insulin
Responses to Orally Administered Simple and Complex
Carbohydrates.*

almost no fat! When a potato is processed into potato chips, it
becomes more than forty percent (40%) fat! This processing has
transformed a perfectly nutritious carbohydrate into a **fat chip!**

Studies confirm that the unprocessed carbohydrates like brown rice,
whole grain bread, millet, oatmeal, barley, and starchy vegetables
are converted into glucose which is quickly used as fuel by the
muscles and organs. The remaining glucose is converted to
glycogen and stored as energy in the muscles.[13] The energy
requirement for storing carbohydrates in the muscle is only five to

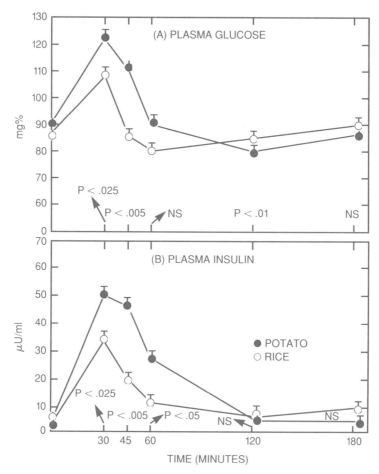

Source: Department of Medicine and Clinical Research Center, Stanford University Medical Center, *Plasma Glucose and Insulin Responses to Orally Administered Simple and Complex Carbohydrates.*

seven percent (5%-7%).[14-15] Complex carbohydrates are not easily converted into fat like the simple carbohydrates.[15-16] **The body requires four times as much energy to convert complex carbohydrate into bodyfat than it does into muscle.** If you had to transport yourself from the first to the sixth floor of an office building, would you take the stairs or the elevator? Most of us would take the elevator because considerably less energy is expended. Your body, like you, will choose the easier way and take the elevator! In studies where 2,000 calories of carbohydrate were eaten at one meal, less than one percent (1%) of the calories was converted into fat![13]

Carbohydrates for Better Thermogenesis

In numerous studies, carbohydrates have been shown to significantly increase the production of heat (thermogenesis) during the process of metabolism.[13, 15, 17, 18] When compared with fats and proteins, the thermogenic effect of carbohydrates is much greater. Because the body is continually producing heat to break down the slowly digesting complex carbohydrates, they are the best time-released fuel to fire up the body's metabolism all day. Even if a person overeats complex carbohydrates, the excess is burned as heat and not stored as fat![17] **That's good news!**

Whole Grains for Weight Loss

Whole grains, are the best starchy carbohydrates for fat loss and weight control. Slowly digesting grains have a stabilizing effect upon glucose and insulin levels which keeps them from being stored as fat.[3, 13] However, in the past eighty years, dietary fat and simple carbohydrates have increased in our diets while grain consumption has declined by forty percent (40%). Replacing fat and simple sugars with whole grains will turn the weight problem in America around.

Many calorie-cutting diets emphasize **cutting fat** without stressing the vital importance of **including grains.** The company to keep is just as important as the company to stay away from! In the next chapter we will examine some of **"Those Incredible Grains."**

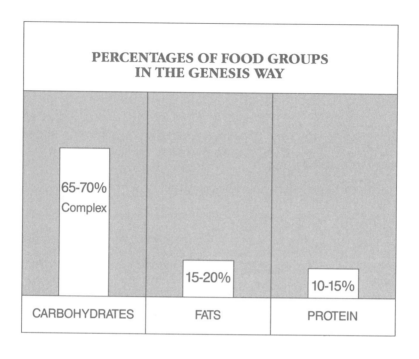

PERCENTAGES OF FOOD GROUPS IN THE GENESIS WAY

65-70%
Complex

15-20%

10-15%

CARBOHYDRATES | FATS | PROTEIN

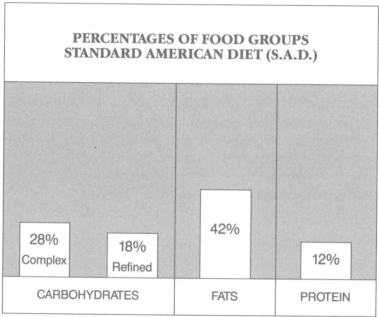

PERCENTAGES OF FOOD GROUPS STANDARD AMERICAN DIET (S.A.D.)

28%
Complex

18%
Refined

42%

12%

CARBOHYDRATES | FATS | PROTEIN

Source: Dietary Goals for the U.S. Select Committee on Nutritional
& Human Needs U.S. Senate.

CHAPTER SEVEN

THOSE INCREDIBLE GRAINS

"There's a great new rice diet that always works -
you use one chopstick."
Red Buttons

Whole grains are the foundation of the Genesis Way of life. They provide the finest complex carbohydrate and fiber available in the entire food chain. They build muscle, increase energy, and fire up your metabolism. They keep us lean and our bodyfat low. Slowly digesting grains are God's natural sugar that provide you with a continuous stream of energy. They are an ideal source of fuel for the brain, nervous system, muscles, hormones, glands and organs.

Thousands of years ago, farming and agriculture developed domesticated cereal grains, vegetables, and fruits that remain in use today. Entire cultures lived on a staple grain product such as rice, millet, lentils or beans. Anthropologists have estimated that some of these grains have been cultivated for thousands of years. Other than tomatoes and coffee, no important new plants have been cultivated in the last two thousand years.

> Rice-12,000 years
> Beans- 9,000 years
> Wheat and Barley-7,000 years

A kernel of grain is made up of three parts: the bran, the endosperm, and the germ. The bran is the outermost part of the grain and the finest source of roughage. It contains vitamins, minerals, and proteins. The endosperm is primarily starch. As it slowly digests, it produces energy in the form of glucose. The germ is rich in protein, polyunsaturated fatty acids, vitamins, and minerals. When grains are "refined" (a polite term for "destroyed"), they are stripped of the bran and the germ. Grains are also composed of "phytic acid" or "phytates." Phytates, found in the outer part of the kernel, protect the grain from decay. Grains should be cooked or sprouted to prevent phytates from pulling minerals, especially calcium, from the body.

MAKE-UP OF A KERNEL OF GRAIN
Oats, brown rice, millet, barley, buckwheat, rye, cornmeal.

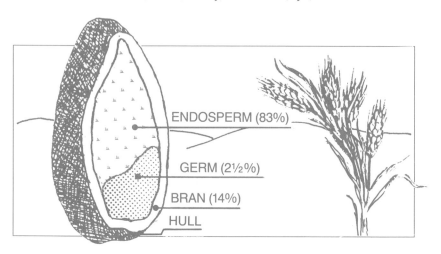

ENDOSPERM (83%)

GERM (2½%)

BRAN (14%)

HULL

TOTAL NUTRIENTS IN A KERNEL OF GRAIN

GERM	BRAN	ENDOSPERM
Thiamine (B^1) Riboflavin (B^2) Pyridoxine (B^6) Protein Pantothenic Acid (B^5) Niacin (B^3) Vitamin E	Pyridoxine (B^6) Pantothenic Acid (B^5) Riboflavin (B^2) Thiamine (B^1) Protein	Starch Traces of Vitamins & Minerals

MINERALS

Calcium	Sulphur	Barium
Iron	Iodine	Silver
Phosophorus	Fluorine	Inositol
Magnesium	Chlorine	Folic Acid
Potassium	Sodium	Choline
Manganese	Silicon	And other trace
Copper	Boron	materials

Source: Nutrition Almanac

Because these truly **incredible** grains are of prime importance to the Genesis Way of life, we will take a brief look at the history of a few of the most beneficial ones. Some of these ancient grains may be new to you. Start eating the familiar ones first, then, when you are feeling leaner and more adventurous, try the new ones!

Amaranth

Amaranth was a daily staple of the Aztec Indians. It is actually not a grain, but a seed. The seeds are about the size of poppy seeds and have a crunchy texture. Amaranth is high in fiber, vitamins A and C, the amino acid lysine, and it is low in gluten. It is sixteen percent (16%) protein and rich in calcium and phosphorous. **Amaranth contains more iron than any other plant!** The leaves can be used as a vegetable and the seeds can be popped like popcorn!

Barley

Barley is one of the oldest cultivated cereals. It probably originated in Africa or Asia. The Egyptians used this valuable food for man and animals as early as 5,000 B.C.E. China began cultivating it about 3,000 B.C.E. Barley was the chief bread ingredient of the Hebrews, Greeks, and Romans. It is mentioned frequently in the Bible and the prophets ate it as their staple food.

Barley was grown in Europe in the Middle Ages and brought to America by the British and the Dutch. The spread of barley to the West was not for food, but rather for making beer. Less than one-tenth of the barley grown in the United States is used for human food.

Barley is a hearty, filling grain. It makes a delicious addition to soups and stews. It can be substituted for rice in most recipes. Barley flour may be used in breads and pancake mixes. It is an excellent source of complete protein, natural sugars and all the essential amino acids. Barley is gluten free and is rich in calcium, iron, thiamin (B1), riboflavin (B2), and niacin (B3).

Buckwheat

Buckwheat was used by the Phoenicians in ancient China. Migrating tribes from Siberia and Manchuria introduced it into

Eastern Europe and the Mediterranean. It is not a grain, but the fruit of a plant. Instead of growing straight and tall like most grains, it grows more like a weed. Buckwheat has heart-shaped leaves and white flowers that attract hungry bees. It can be made into flour for pancakes or eaten as a nutritious gluten-free cereal. Buckwheat contains complete protein, vitamins, and minerals, especially manganese and magnesium. It is high in **rutin**, a bioflavinoid, found to be helpful in lowering blood pressure, aiding the circulatory system and easing painful hemorrhoids. Buckwheat is one of those foods an individual either loves or hates! The Jewish people eat a traditional buckwheat dish known as **Kasha.**

Corn (Maize)

According to archaeologists, corn grew wild in southern Mexico nine thousand years ago! The Indians of Central and South America have been using corn for centuries. The Mayas, Incas, and Aztecs worshipped the plant as a god. The American Indians thought so highly of the grain that it became a part of their religious practices. The American Indians called corn: "Seed of Seeds," "Sacred Mother," and "Blessed Daughter."

Corn is very economical since it yields three times as much harvest per acre as wheat. Corn is a high protein seed that is actually a grass. Yellow corn is preferred because of its abundant amount of vitamin A. It also contains the largest amount of energy producing starch. Its germ is particularly rich in unsaturated fatty acids. Corn is not rich in minerals or the B vitamins.

Chief Varieties of Corn

Flint Corn -   very hardy, shiny grain with a good percentage of protein content.

Dent Corn -   more starchy than flint and this variety predominates U.S. "corn belt".

Flown Corn -   usually white and the starch is so soft that it easily forms a paste when mixed with water.

Sweet Corn -   the variety referred to as "Indian Corn" or "corn on the cob".

Popcorn -   the popping action turns the grain **inside out!** When the water contained in the center of the grain is heated, it builds up such pressure that it explodes! Use "air" popped popcorn when possible.

Millet
Millet has the ability to support human life in the absence of all other foods. This makes it unique among the grains. Its name is derived from a Latin word meaning "a thousand" because of its numerous seeds. This grain has been found in the pyramids and tombs of the ancient Egyptians. Over 2,500 years ago, Pythagoras, the Greek philosopher, encouraged his followers to eat millet to improve their health and vitality. In the Bible, the prophet Ezekiel was told by God to make bread out of millet and other grains.

Millet is native to eastern Asia and is a staple of northern China today. It is also the staple food of the Hunzakuts, a culture renowned for their superior health, virility, and long life. Many of them live to be a hundred years old! The Georgian people of Russia, are another long-lived group who eat millet regularly and are reported to be free of heart disease, cancer, diabetes, and arthritis. Unfortunately, millet is used mostly for birdseed in the United States.

Millet has all the essential amino acids comparable to meat or dairy products. It contains all the minerals and is especially rich in calcium, magnesium, potassium, iron, and florine. Millet is rich in the B vitamins, thiamin and riboflavin, as well as vitamin A and vitamin C. It also contains choline which helps to keep cholesterol levels low. Since millet is an alkaline food, unlike most grains, it is well tolerated by individuals with over-acid and ulcerative conditions. Millet, according to nutritionist Dr. Paavo Airola, is not fattening because its alkaline properties tend to counteract fat building in the body. Millet is a high fiber carbohydrate that is easily digested and can be substituted for rice in any recipe.

Oats

This grain was developed around 2,500 B.C.E. in northern Africa, the Near East and Russia. Today, oats are a staple food in Scotland, Ireland, and northern England. In the United States, oats, like millet, are used mostly to feed animals.

An oat groat, the whole grain, is very soft and can be crushed easily with a rolling pin. Breaking down the grain in this manner makes it easy to cook. Old-fashioned rolled oats, not the quick-cooking variety, are very nutritious. Oatflakes are a popular ingredient in many "health" products. Oat flour is an excellent ingredient in breads and muffins. Of all the grains, oats are the most acidic. They also contain a high amount of gluten. The bran of oats is an excellent source of fiber that is beneficial in relieving constipation and removing excess cholesterol. Oats are a good source of B vitamins, protein, calcium, and iodine. The iodine content of oats is helpful for a slow-working thyroid. Oats provide energy and stamina by helping to regulate blood glucose levels. **People, as well as horses, will develop endurance and strength by eating oats regularly!**

Quinoa

Quinoa, pronounced "keen-wa", means "mother" or "mother grain." The Academy of Science calls quinoa, "the best source of protein in the vegetable kingdom." Quinoa is a grain-like seed from a fruit found in the South American mountains. It is a member of the same family as spinach, beets, chard, and lamb's quarter. Quinoa is a high source of B vitamins, iron, fiber, calcium, and phosphorus. There is a naturally bitter coating of "saponins" that acts as a built-in pest control for the seeds. In order to remove this coating, the quinoa must be rinsed 3-5 times. It cooks like rice.

Rice

Rice has been a staple food of Asians and Orientals since 3,000 B.C.E. This grain was first cultivated in India. The expansion of Buddhism eventually spread cultivated rice throughout China, Japan, and Asia. Today, rice is the staple food crop for over half the world's population. During most of the year, rice plants must be under one to eight inches of water. Then the fields are drained and the grain is picked. Approximately 200 billion pounds of rice are produced in the world annually. The United States grows only one percent (1%) of the world crop. The average Oriental eats four hundred pounds of rice a year while Americans eat less than ten pounds a year!

Unprocessed rice is naturally brown and highly nutritious. There are two major varieties, short and long grain. Brown rice contains about ten percent (10%) protein, seven percent (7%) fat, and eighty-three percent (83%) carbohydrates. Ironically, only the poorest people in the Orient eat this type of rice while it is a status symbol to have the white, polished type of rice. After the husk, bran, and germ are removed by milling, the white starchy substance that remains is polished. Beri-beri is a disease associated with those people who subsist on a diet of polished rice. The cause of beri-beri is a deficiency of B-1 or thiamine which is lost during the polishing process. Rice flour can be added to bread recipes in place of wheat flour. This is especially important for those who are allergic to wheat. Rice can also be added to soups and stews or eaten as a side dish. Basmati brown rice is a nutty, non-gummy rice grown in Texas. Incredibly, there are 7,000 varieties of rice!

Rye
Rye was discovered in Turkey and Greece. The Europeans in the Middle Ages harvested wild rye while gathering other crops. It was a weed that grew along side the cultivated grains. Rye is the heartiest of all the grains. It is high in protein, low in gluten and possesses a strong flavor. Rye has the highest amount of the amino acid lysine. This hearty grain can be ground into flour to produce rye or pumpernickel breads. Rye can be used in place of rice or it can also be flaked like oats, which makes it easier and faster to cook.

Spelt
Spelt is an ancient grain mentioned in the Bible. Allergic individuals often tolerate it well because of its digestibility. Spelt is a high gluten product which contains more vitamin B1 and B2 than any other grain. It is an excellent source of valuable minerals and contains all the essential amino acids. Spelt aids digestion, promotes elimination, and helps the immune system. Spelt flour can be used in recipes calling for whole wheat flour.

Teff

Because teff is the smallest grain in the world, the word teff means "lost." One hundred and fifty grains of teff weigh the same as a single grain of wheat! Ounce for ounce, teff has more nutrient-rich bran, germ, iron, calcium, and potassium, than any other grain in the world. Teff contains substantial amounts of protein. It is a gluten-free, easily digested grain containing both soluble and insoluble fiber. Teff can be used to make flatbreads, cakes, cookies, soups, stews, stir-fry, casseroles, and puddings.

Wheat

Wheat is the most widely grown cereal crop in the world. It was first cultivated in Iraq. Wheat comes in many forms: wheat berries, grits, cream of wheat (no bran), puffed (no nothin'), bulgar, shredded, flakes, gluten flour, germ, cracked, rolled, durum (for pastas), mush, and wheat grass. This popular grain is high in protein, essential minerals, B vitamins, and vitamin E. Hard wheat has a very high gluten content which helps make bread rise. Soft wheat has less gluten and is more suitable in baking cakes, pie crusts, muffins, and biscuits. Gluten is a sticky, tough, protein that forms mucous and coats the villi of the intestines. If the villi become heavily coated with gluten, nutrient absorption can be affected. Wheat can cause constipation, allergies, bloating and even weight gain. Alternating whole wheat with other grain choices will reduce its allergic reactions.

Wild Rice

Wild rice is not a grain at all! This rare aquatic grass seed is grown and harvested in the Great Lakes region of the United States. It must be harvested by hand from canoes, which accounts for its high price tag! Wild rice is high in fiber, low in fat, and is a good source of protein, B vitamins, and essential minerals. Mix it half and half with brown rice for a delicious combination.

Conclusion

Whole grains keep your tummy full, bowels moving, energy high and blood sugar stable. If that does not get you excited, remember this last fact. **Whole grains are very low in fat!** They are unequaled as a treasure chest of vitality and long-lasting energy! Eating these incredible grains 2 to 3 times a day will produce optimum results.

42

WATER EACH DAY TO KEEP FAT AWAY

"Oh that this too too solid flesh
would melt, thaw, and resolve itself into dew."
William Shakespeare

Did you ever stop to think that every glass of water you drink contains molecules that have existed since the earth was formed? The quantity of water on earth is limited. We cannot manufacture "new" water therefore we must recycle and reuse it. Next to air, water is the most essential substance the body needs in order to maintain life. The body is between fifty to sixty percent (50%-60%) water and requires 4-6 pints of fluid daily. This fluid is obtained not only from water, but also from various foods and drinks. Drinking sufficient water helps you maintain a youthful complexion, while drinking too little water can actually cause the skin to wrinkle. You may not consider water as an important nutrient, but it is. Virtually every function in your body requires water.

Water is a catalyst in losing weight and keeping it off
1. Water helps maintain muscle tone; and therefore it also helps prevent "sagging" skin which can follow weight loss. It leaves the skin looking clear, tight, and resilient. It also lubricates your joints and helps prevent dehydration of all cells.
2. Water helps rid the body of waste products via the kidneys and the skin.
3. Sufficient water drinking will keep the bowel moist and help prevent constipation. Retention of extra waste products also adds to excess weight.
4. Water prevents water retention. Water retention is a result of inadequate water consumption. If the body is properly "watered," it would not need to "hold on" to extracellular fluids. Retained water shows up as excess weight. To rid the body of excess water you must drink more water. **Water**

Percentage of Water in the Human Body

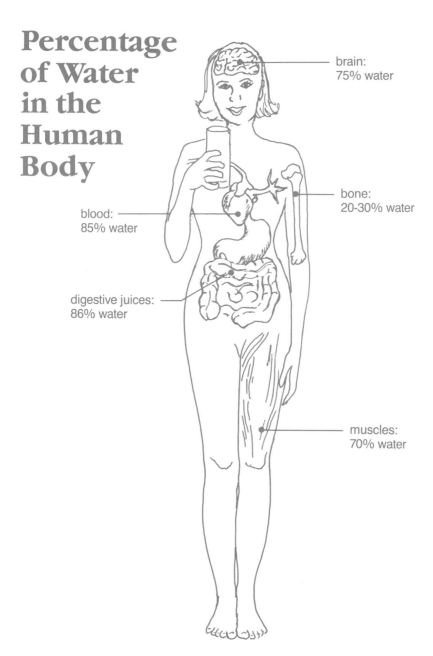

brain:
75% water

bone:
20-30% water

blood:
85% water

digestive juices:
86% water

muscles:
70% water

The average body contains a total of 96 pints of water. Sixty-four pints are found inside the body's cells, with the remainder outside the cells—in the blood, lymph fluid, and digestive juices.

Source: V. Hegarty, *Decisions in Nutrition* (New York: Times Mirror Publishing, 1988).

5. Water rids the body of salt accumulation. It will dilute excess salt and flush it out through the kidneys.
6. Since the brain is seventy-five percent (75%) water, insufficient water can lead to frequent headaches and dizziness.
7. Water suppresses the appetite naturally. A certain amount of hunger is thirst.
8. Water helps mobilize bodyfat. Drinking insufficient amounts of water forces the liver to take on part of the elimination that the kidneys would normally do. The liver helps mobilize stored fat to be burned in the muscle unless this activity is slowed when it is forced to help the kidneys.

The body loses approximately ten cups (80 oz.) of fluid per day. The best way to monitor water requirements is not by thirst alone. Many people are not thirsty, especially overweight people. They tend to mistake thirst for hunger. The best guide to your water needs is to notice the color of the urine. If the urine is dark, it means the kidneys were forced to concentrate the waste in a smaller volume of urine. Pale or clear urine indicates good hydration. **The Genesis Way of life suggests a minimum of six, eight ounce glasses of water a day.** Try to drink thirty minutes before or after a main meal and between meals. The habit of drinking with meals can dilute stomach juices and cause poor digestion in some people.

Remember that your kidneys are a little larger than your ears and should not be overloaded with more than eight ounces of fluid at one time. When water tends to go right through the body, it can indicate a lack of sufficient muscle. The overweight have less capacity to keep water in the tissues because of a lower percentage of lean muscle. A weak bladder can be the result of insufficient water intake.

What is the Best Water?
Next to distilled rain water, the purest water available is steam distilled water. Another pure water is "low sodium" spring water. Several companies offer bottled water. However, be sure to check them out thoroughly. Soft water is not recommended because of the sodium used to process the water. In the home, water filtration

the sodium used to process the water. In the home, water filtration systems such as reverse osmosis and multi-filtered units are worth looking into. Tap water is not recommended. The water we drink helps preserve, nourish, and cleanse our entire body from the brain to the tips of the toes. The Genesis Way encourages developing the positive habit of drinking plenty of pure water throughout the day. I'll drink (water) to that!

CHAPTER NINE

CHOOSE LIFE!

"Behold, I set before you today life and good, death and evil, ...
therefore, choose life, that you and your descendents may live;"
Deuteronomy 30: 15,19

THE GENESIS WAY PRINCIPLES

You have come to where you are today as a result of past choices.
What you will become tomorrow is the result of today's choices.
Choose life today, the Genesis Way!

A. Eat often to lose.
Eating frequently during the day stokes the fire of thermogenesis in
the body and increases your metabolism. On the other hand,
infrequent eating slows your metabolism. **Use it (metabolism) or
lose it!**

B. Choose thermogenic foods.
The type of calories you eat is just as important to increase your
metabolism as how often you eat. Compared with fats and
proteins, starchy carbohydrates, especially grains, are far better at
producing heat (thermogenesis) which boosts metabolism. The
steady stream of energy these thermogenic foods provide insures
that the body will burn calories all day long! They are the preferred
fuel to fire up our fat-burning furnace!

C. Forget calories! Think fat!
All calories are not created equal. Ninety-seven percent (97%) of
the fat you eat is stored as bodyfat, whereas, only one percent (1%)
of the starchy carbohydrates you eat is stored as bodyfat.
Therefore just counting calories is not the solution to your weight
problems. Instead, if you concentrate on limiting fat grams, you can
watch the inches and bodyfat disappear! The issue is not just being
overweight, it is being overfat!

D. Increase muscle mass to burn fat.

We need to decrease our bodyfat and increase our muscle mass. The muscle of the body is the primary fat-burning furnace. **Ninety percent (90%) of our metabolism takes place in our muscles.** [1] Complex carbohydrates are not easily stored as fat and provide food for the muscles. Eating lots of grains and engaging in strength training exercises will build the muscle we need to burn fat.

E. Drink water to satisfy hunger.

A certain amount of hunger is really thirst. Drinking plenty of water suppresses the appetite naturally. Water is the finest thirst and hunger quencher in the world! Therefore, water is a catalyst in losing weight. Drink a minimum of six, eight ounce glasses a day.

F. Avoid simple carbohydrates

Simple carbohydrates like refined sugar and fruit juices increase the appetite for more simple sugars. Foods that contain simple sugars often have high amounts of fat in them and fat is easily converted into bodyfat. The fructose contained in fruit and fruit-juice sweetened products is also converted into fat. In order to lose bodyfat and control hunger, simple carbohydrates should be kept to a minimum.

Where to Begin

First you must ask yourself, **"What is my current percent of bodyfat?"** The answer to this question will help you chart your progress. Health clubs and sports medicine facilities will usually measure your bodyfat percentage for a fee. There are four basic ways to measure bodyfat: underwater weighing, skinfold calipers, bioelectric impedance and infrared interactance. All of these techniques have their advantages and disadvantages. The skinfold calipers are probably the most common method and also the most economical. You may order your own, inexpensive, easy-to-use bodyfat calipers from the Genesis Way by calling 1-800-GEN-LIFE, 1-800-436-5433.

Breaking the Fat Barrier

MEASUREMENTS	BEGINNING	1ST MONTH	2ND MONTH	3RD MONTH	4TH MONTH
% Body Fat					
Neck					
Upper Arm					
Chest/Bust					
Waist					
Hips					
Thigh					
Calf					

Desired Bodyfat

Optimal weight relates more to bodyfat than to pounds. The correct percentage of bodyfat for your age found in the chart below applies to an average person. Athletes and those who exercise regularly should subtract two to three percent (2%-3%). The average range for men is between fifteen to twenty percent (l5%-20%) bodyfat. For women, the average range is between nineteen to twenty-four percent (19%-24%).

Correct Bodyfat Percentage

Age	Males	Females
16-19	15%	19%
20-29	16%	20%
30-39	17%	21%
40-49	18%	22%
50-59	19%	23%
60+	20%	24%

(data-Dr. David Parker, physiologist)

Desired Body Weight

Once you have determined your correct bodyfat percentage, you are ready to compute your desired body weight. The following computation for desired body weight is taken from <u>EXERCISE PHYSIOLOGY</u> by McArdle, Katch and Katch.[2]

Suppose a twenty-seven year old woman, who weighs 150 pounds with thirty percent (30%) bodyfat, wants to find out what her **desired weight** should be. First, she would determine the optimum bodyfat percentage for her age, which is twenty percent (20%). Then, she would do the following calculations to compute her desired weight:

l. Current Weight X Current Bodyfat = Fat Weight
    150 pounds   X   30%   =   45 pounds

2. Current Weight - Fat Weight = Lean Body Weight
    150 pounds   -   45 pounds   =   105 pounds

3. $\dfrac{\text{Lean body weight}}{1.00 - \text{optimal bodyfat}}$　　=　　Desired Body Weight

$\dfrac{105 \text{ pounds}}{1.00 - .20}$

$\dfrac{105 \text{ pounds}}{.80 \text{ pounds}}$　　=　　**131 pounds**
(Desired Body Weight)

4. Current Body Weight - Desired Body Weight = **Desired Fat Loss**
    150 pounds　　-　　131 pounds　　=　　**19 pounds**

This hypothetical twenty-seven year old woman, with an optimum bodyfat of twenty percent (20%), should actually weigh 131 pounds! When you compute your desired body weight, you may think the weight is either too high or too low. But remember, you are not only losing bodyfat, you are gaining lean muscle. You will look much leaner than you do right now by the time you reach your bodyfat goal. So don't judge your desired body weight until you arrive at the new you. When you look in the mirror a few months from now, you will like what you see!

Your Fat Budget
The total number of fat grams that you eat each day in order to maintain a lean body is your Fat Budget. Women should have a Fat Budget of **33 grams** a day and men **53 grams** a day. A **minimum** of three meals and three snacks should be eaten each day. You are free to choose any combination of meals and snacks you desire, as long as you stay within your Fat Budget. Your Fat Budget will also help you make wise food choices at restaurants and grocery stores.

Fat Budget Should Consist of Essential Fats
Fats are portrayed as "bad for us," and yet we cannot live without them. Sufficient amounts of essential fatty acids are needed for optimum health and weight control. Maintaining adequate levels of dietary fats enable the body to assimilate certain fat soluble vitamins such as vitamins A, D, E, F, and K. The Surgeon General's Report on Nutrition and Health(1988) sums up the need for adequate fat in the diet: "Adults need a minimum daily intake of

15 to 25 grams of fat to meet these necessities."[30] Obviously, fat must not be totally eliminated from our diets. **The essential fatty acids contained in fish and vegetable oils should make up most of our Fat Budget.**

How to Eat
There are 3 types of eaters: Grabbers, Gorgers, and Grazers!

Grabbers are people who eat on the run. They eat when they have time and what they eat is of little concern to them. Their food choice is usually something quick. Grabbers are not particularly interested in food because other things are more important. They "grab a bite," before rushing off to their next appointment.

Gorgers eat large amounts of food at one or two sittings. They usually miss breakfast, but make up for the lost calories sometime later in the day. They may eat 1,000 to 3,000 calories at a meal and then not eat for many hours. This pattern of large, infrequent meals sets the stage for the body to store the excess calories as fat. Gorgers tend to gain weight easily with this pattern and usually have accompanying digestive discomforts like bloating, gas, heart burn, sleepiness, foggy-headedness, and fatigue after these substantial meals. The sumo wrestlers of Japan are a prime example of how to gain weight by gorging. Although their diet consists of rice, fish, vegetables and very little fat, how and when they eat is the secret to their tremendous size. Sumo wrestlers deliberately "starve" themselves all day and then eat one or two big meals in the evening in order to gain weight![4]

Grazers eat 6 to 8 small meals a day and usually do not have weight problems. By eating frequently, they keep the thermogenic effect of food stoking their metabolism all day long. Children are natural grazers. They eat a little bit here and a little bit there, until a well-meaning, though misguided, parent refuses to let them eat between meals. Studies clearly demonstrate that eating several small meals a day does not cause excessive accumulations of fat. Eating the same amount of food in only one or two meals can cause more fat storage.[5-6] **Let's hear it for the grazers! They eat the Genesis Way!**

When to Eat

In order to break the fat barrier, a person must eat a minimum of **six times** each day. This might be difficult at first, especially for chronic dieters. But remember, **food is fuel** and the body must have adequate calories in order to operate properly. Chronic dieters eat too little and they eat the wrong kinds of food. Dieting leaves a person tired and their metabolism sluggish. The latest research shows that losing bodyfat and building lean muscle depends on eating more calories, not less. We were created to eat good food. The Genesis Way of life stresses healthy food and plenty of it! Schedule your meals and snacks as follows:

1. **Morning breakfast**
2. **Mid-morning snack**
3. **Mid-day meal**
4. **Mid-afternoon snack**
5. **Evening meal**
6. **Evening snack**

Most of us live according to a schedule, even if we do not think so. We **make** time to work, time for appointments, time to watch television, time to go out to dinner, and time to go to the movies. We need to **make** time for meals and snacks as well. There are three good reasons for scheduling times to eat often during the day:

1. **Eating frequently during the day boosts our metabolism.**
Our body is a furnace that requires food as its fuel. Every time we eat, we raise the heat of our body in order to metabolize the food. Cutting calories and skipping meals lowers the metabolism. By eating thermogenic foods more often, we will speed up our metabolism and not store fat!

2. **Eating often insures a stable blood sugar and energy level.**
When we eat complex carbohydrates throughout the day we provide our body with a continuous supply of glucose energy. Eating these nutritious foods restores energy and vitality, while skipping meals leads to fatigue and mood swings.

3.   Frequent eating burns fat while infrequent eating builds fat!

Remember the sumo wrestlers of Japan? Their gain is our loss if we do not emulate their eating patterns of one or two big meals a day. Eat like grazing children and you will not store fat.

Eat Breakfast and Increase Your Metabolism

Some people trying to "diet" say they are afraid to eat breakfast because they will be hungry all day. The thermogenic effect of eating breakfast **"jump starts"** our metabolism in the morning and eating frequently will keep it going all day. Studies indicate the overweight rarely eat a breakfast meal.[7] **A recent study at Vanderbilt confirmed that obese breakfast-skippers who began to eat breakfast lost seventeen pounds in twelve weeks.**[8] Eating large dinners late in the evening will cause weight gain, but eating large breakfasts will not! Eating breakfast fires-up the body's metabolism to burn fat all day! Some people say that they are not hungry in the morning. The reason for their lack of appetite is that they eat large meals late at night. If you are one of these people, follow this simple rule: Never eat more at dinner than you ate for breakfast! If you did not eat breakfast, do not eat dinner! I guarantee that you will be hungry the next morning!

Healthiest cultures on earth

Most nutrition controversy would end if nutritionists would stop promoting their own personal dietary ideas and study the dietary patterns of cultures renown for their healthy, disease-free lifestyles. These healthy lifestyles enable certain cultures to live free of cancer, heart disease, arthritis, PMS, strokes, and diabetes, just to name a few problems common to many Americans. Such extraordinary cultures include the traditional Japanese and Chinese, the Equadorian Vilcabambas, the Pakastani Hunzakuts, the traditional Bulgarians, the Yucatan and Chihuahua Indians of Mexico, and the Abkhazians of Georgian Russia.

Healthy Cultures

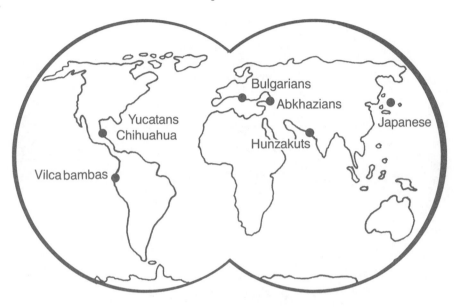

Although scattered throughout the world, these cultures have strikingly similar eating patterns. Their diets are high in complex carbohydrates and fiber, moderate in protein, and low in fat, especially cholesterol and saturated fat. All of these cultures are grazers rather than grabbers or gorgers, eating several small meals a day. Last, but not least, in all these healthy cultures there is virtually no obesity, despite the unrestricted caloric intake.

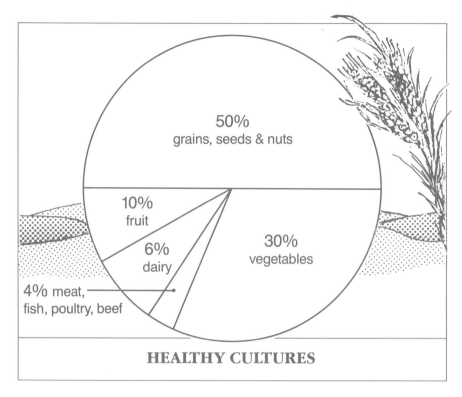

50%
grains, seeds & nuts

10%
fruit

6%
dairy

30%
vegetables

4% meat,
fish, poultry, beef

HEALTHY CULTURES

You only have four simple rules to remember:

1. **Stay within your Fat Budget**
2. **Gradually increase the frequency of meals and snacks**
3. **Eat grains two or three times a day**
4. **Drink six, eight ounce glasses of pure water a day**

The Genesis Way of life will dramatically boost your metabolism and help you break the fat barrier. The permanent loss of bodyfat and the building of lean muscle does not lie in the restriction of dietary fat alone, but in eating the grains that fuel thermogenesis. Since you gained weight over a period of time, you must lose it over a period of time. A healthy, safe and permanent weight loss would be one to two pounds per week. If you are faithful to this lifestyle, you should see "measurable" results within twelve weeks. As you choose life The Genesis Way, you will drop several clothes sizes while reducing your bodyfat and increasing your lean muscle. How exciting your future is The Genesis Way.

There's only one way...The Genesis Way!

CHAPTER TEN

EATING THE GENESIS WAY

"The two biggest sellers in any bookstore are cookbooks and the diet books. The cookbooks tell you how to prepare the food and the diet books tell you how not to eat any of it."
Andy Rooney

This section of **BREAKING THE FAT BARRIER** answers the question, **"What do I eat, and how do I prepare it?"** The Genesis Way of life is simple and easy, whether you are eating at home or in a restaurant. You will **never** have to count calories again - only fat grams. For your convenience, fat grams have been calculated for the recipes and snacks in this section. When eating out, refer to the companion booklet, **Countdown to Breaking the Fat Barrier,** to calculate fat grams. You are **FREE** to choose **any** combination of meals and snacks, as long as you stay within your **Fat Budget.**

FAT BUDGETS

WOMEN: 33 GRAMS PER DAY

MEN: 53 GRAMS PER DAY

UNLIMITED FOODS
The unlimited foods contribute very little fat to your **Fat Budget.**
You may use them **freely** in your meal plans.

Beans
Egg Whites or Egg Beaters (liquid egg substitute)
Fat Free Snacks (except fruit)
Fat Free Soups
Fresh Lemon and Lime Juice
Grains
Legumes
Spices
Vegetables
Water: At least (6) 8 oz. glasses (Distilled or Spring Water)

LIMITED FOODS
Any or all of the limited foods may be used in your meal plans as
part of your **Fat Budget.** Stay within the following limits:

Almonds	6 per snack = 3.6 grams of fat
Almond Butter	1 tablespoon = 9.5 grams of fat
Chicken (no skin)	2 meals per week
Eggs	2 whole eggs per week
Fish (no shellfish)	3 meals per week (Salmon as one meal)
Fruit	1 apple per day for the first 90 days. After 90 days, 2 fruits per day.
Pasta	1 meal per week (no egg or ramen noodles)

Potatoes	Sweet: 2 meals per week
	White or Red: 1 meal per week
Red Meat	1 meal per month
Turkey (no skin)	2 meals per week
Vegetable Oil	1 tablespoon per day
	(Olive, Safflower, Canola)

ESSENTIAL FATS
All types of oil have 14 grams of fat per tablespoon

Almonds	6 almonds = 3.6 grams of fat
Canola Oil	use for cooking, salads, may add to grains
Fish	see Limited Foods
Olive Oil	use for cooking, salads, may add to grains
Safflower Oil	not for cooking: it will turn rancid, refrigerate
Sesame Oil	excellent for stir-frying
Cooking Spray	1 spray = 1 gram of fat

FAT FREE SNACKS

Apples	Rice Cakes
Apple Butter	Salsa
Bagels	Soups
Cereals	Unsulphured Raisins
Crackers	Vegetables
Currents	Whole Grain Breads
Pretzels	Yogurt

SWEET TREATS
Once a Week

Banana
Frozen Yogurt
Fruit Juice Sweetened Fat Free Cookies
Honey Maid Graham Crackers

COOKING WHOLE GRAINS

Whole grains can be cooked in a glass or stainless steel pan on your stove.

1) For every cup of dry grain you wish to cook, use 2.5 parts distilled or spring water. (see chart below)

2) **Grains must be thoroughly washed before cooking.** Use a wire mesh strainer to rinse measured grain.

3) In a pan add water and washed grain. Cover pan with a tight fitting lid and bring to a boil. Reduce heat to low and cook until liquid is absorbed. (See chart below for cooking times) Do not remove cover or stir grain while cooking.

4) When done, remove from heat and let stand 5-10 minutes. Fluff with a fork and serve.

GRAIN YIELD CHART

GRAIN	DRY	COOKED	COOKING TIME
Barley (pearled)	1 cup	9 cups	10-12 Minutes
Brown Rice	1 cup	3 cups	40-45 Minutes
Millet	1 cup	5 cups	35-40 Minutes
Oats	1 cup	2 cups	5-10 Minutes
Quinoa	1 cup	3 cups	15-20 Minutes

If you are using an electric rice cooker, follow the manufacturer's directions. A rice cooker should have either a teflon coated or stainless steel liner. Avoid brands that are lined only with aluminum.

SAUTEING WITH LESS OIL

Our culture is so dependent upon the use of oil and butter for cooking that we have little to no idea of what food tastes like without it! One of the most important changes you will make is cooking with less fat! Try these condiments in **addition** to a **small** amount of oil for sauteing and stir-fry fun! They may also be used instead of the oil.

De-Fatted Chicken Broth   **Lemon or Lime Juice**
Pure Water   **Salsa**
Soy Sauce (reduced sodium)   **Tomato Juice**
Vegetable Cooking Spray   **Worcestershire Sauce**

BROWNING ONIONS AND VEGETABLES WITHOUT FAT

Browned onions make other vegetables taste so good because they have a delicious, rich flavor. You can brown them without using *ANY FAT!*

1 1/2 cups chopped onions
3 cups of water
non-stick frying pan
vegetable cooking spray

Add the onions and 1 cup of water to the nonstick frying pan and cook over medium heat stirring occasionally. Continue to stir until the onions begin to thicken on the pan bottom, and the water begins to disappear. Add another 1/2 cup of water, and continue to stir, loosening the browned bits from the bottom of the pan. Cook until the water disappears again. Repeat this process as many times as necessary to give you the rich brown color you like. You can also use this method to brown garlic, potatoes, carrots and other vegetables.

HOMEMADE DE-FATTED CHICKEN BROTH

8 cups of spring or distilled water
3 lbs. of chicken parts (wings, backs, necks, ribs)
1 large yellow onion, cut into wedges
2 stalks of celery, cut into chunks
1 large carrot, cut into chunks
1 tsp. parsley flakes
1 bay leaf
1/4 tsp. black pepper
mesh strainer, small holes

Add first 8 ingredients to a large pot, and bring to a boil. Reduce heat, cover and simmer for 2-3 hours or until the chicken parts are separated from their bones. Remove the bones, and strain the broth through a mesh strainer into a large bowl or pot. Cover the bowl or pot, and refrigerate until the fat congeals and forms a hard layer at the top. Skim off the fat layer and discard. Refrigerate or freeze the broth for later use.

SMART TIPS: Freeze some of the de-fatted broth in an ice cube tray, and when frozen, store the cubes in a freezer bag. Use one or more cubes in recipes calling for de-fatted broth. (Most ice cube trays hold approximately 2 TBS. per section). **If you prefer, you can purchase canned de-fatted chicken broth in most supermarkets.**

A WORD ON DAIRY PRODUCTS

Dairy products, especially cow's milk, are the second leading cause of allergies in the United States. Some people are allergic to the protein in cow's milk called **casein.** Casein helps a calf grow into a 1000 pound animal! The primary protein in mother's milk is lactoalbumin, not casein. Mother's milk, not cow's milk is the perfect food for infants!

Lactose intolerance is another type of allergic reaction to milk. This type of allergic reaction is caused by not having a sufficient amount of **lactase**. Lactase is the human enzyme that digests the milk sugar, lactose. Lactose intolerance can cause bloating, gas, cramps, mucus buildup, constipation, and or diarrhea.

Allergies to cow's milk can continue throughout adulthood and apply to ALL milk based dairy products! For those who **can tolerate** cow's milk, choose low-fat or nonfat varieties.

TYPE OF MILK (1 CUP)	GRAMS OF FAT
Whole Milk	8.5
2 % Milk	5.3
1 % Milk	2.5
Skim Milk	0.4

YOGURT

Unlike other dairy products, yogurt digests itself because it contains friendly bacteria (lactobacillus bulgaricus and streptococcus thermophilus). These friendly organisms are found in most yogurt and they create lactase, the enzyme which digests milk sugar (lactose). **Yogurt does not cause allergic reactions in most milk allergic people.**

Choose low-fat or nonfat varieties. Whenever possible choose plain yogurt to avoid unwanted sugars. Adding fresh fruit to plain yogurt will provide taste, vitamins, minerals and extra fiber.

BUTTER

Butter, either lightly salted or unsalted has 11 grams of fat per tablespoon! Butter is better than margarine, but not as healthy as olive or canola oil.

CHEESE

The Genesis Way recommends avoiding cheese whenever possible. All types of cheese can be constipating, mucus forming and allergy producing, even without the fat!

Recipes For
Breaking The Fat Barrier

The following recipes were selected because:

THEY ARE LOW-FAT AND TASTE GOOD!
Each recipe has been given the **nutritional seal of approval** and has **passed the taste test** by the most serious panel of judges.....husbands, children, housewives and singles!

THEY ARE GOOD FOR YOU!
The **thermogenic** foods from the earth are **the** foods of **The Genesis Way.** They will fill you up, satisfy you, and **will turn your body into a fat-burning furnace!**

THEY ARE EASY TO PREPARE!
Making a lifestyle change does not have to be complicated. Each recipe has been designed to use the minimum number of ingredients and take the least amount of preparation time.

THEY OFFER YOU LOTS OF VARIETY!
Each recipe section offers you a variety of choices so you will not get bored. You can make simple changes that suit your taste and your family's.

THEY ARE BUDGET MINDED!
These recipes will help you and your family conserve food dollars because they are made with pure, whole ingredients which do not require fancy packaging and processing costs.

BREAKFAST MEALS

	GRAMS OF FAT	PAGE #
Breakfast Bars	3.7	68
Creamy Apple Porridge	1.8	68
Eggs and Wild Rice	less than one	69
Kellogg's Nutri-Grain	1.0	69
Millet Fruit Pudding	5.5	70
Oatmeal Breakfast Muffins	2.7	71
Orange Pancakes	2.6	72
Outstanding Oats	6.3	72
Raisin Breakfast Grain	1.5	73
Raisins and Spice Oats	1.8	73
Rice Pudding	3.0	74
Spanish Omelet	13.1	74
Very Easy French Toast	2.2	75
Weekend Breakfast Quiche	6.0	76

BREAKFAST BARS
3.7 grams of fat per serving

1 1/2 cup rolled oats, uncooked
3/4 cup chopped dates
1/2 tsp. grated orange rind
1 tsp. cinnamon
1/2 tsp. sea salt
1/4 cup chopped walnuts or pecans
1/4 cup water
1/2 cup unsweetened apple sauce
1/4 cup nonfat plain yogurt
1 shredded, medium raw apple
vegetable cooking spray

Combine all ingredients in a large bowl and press together. Let stand at room temperature for 10 minutes. Press mixture into an 8" x 8" baking dish sprayed with vegetable cooking spray. Bake at 375 degrees for 20 to 25 minutes. Loosen loaf with spatula and cut into 6-8 bars while warm. Serve with a little plain low-fat yogurt if desired. Makes a great lunchbox snack! *SIX SERVINGS*

CREAMY APPLE PORRIDGE
1.8 grams of fat per serving

1/2 unpeeled apple, coarsely chopped
1/3 cup uncooked rolled oats
3/4 cup water
1/4 tsp. cinnamon

Place apple in a blender and process on low speed until smooth. Combine applesauce with the oats and water in a medium saucepan. Add cinnamon, stir and cook about 5 to 10 minutes, until the oatmeal is creamy. Top with a spoonful of unsweetened applesauce, nonfat plain yogurt or a few raisins if desired. *ONE SERVING*

EGGS AND WILD RICE
less than one gram of fat per serving

one cup egg beaters
1/4 cup cooked wild rice
1/8 cup skim milk
1/2 tsp. Worcestershire sauce
dash of sea salt
dash of hot sauce
vegetable cooking spray

Combine all ingredients in a large bowl; beat with a fork or whisk until ingredients are well blended. Coat a large non-stick skillet with vegetable cooking spray. Place skillet over medium-low heat until pan is hot. Pour in egg mixture. When eggs begin to set, stir gently to allow uncooked portions to flow underneath. Cook until done. *ONE SERVING*

KELLOGG'S NUTRI-GRAIN WHEAT CEREAL
1 gram of fat per serving

To 3/4 cup packaged **KELLOGG'S Nutri-Grain Wheat Cereal** in a bowl add:
1 teaspoon currants or 2 teaspoons raisins and
1 cup nonfat milk

Serving ideas: add 1/2 sliced apple, 1/2 sliced banana or 2-3 sliced strawberries. *ONE SERVING*

MILLET FRUIT PUDDING
5.5 grams of fat per serving

1/2 cup canned crushed pineapple, juice reserved
1/2 tsp. vanilla extract
2-3 fresh strawberries, sliced
3/4 cup hot, freshly cooked millet
1/2 cup water
dash sea salt
1 TBS. raisins
6 raw almonds, diced

Place a layer of sliced strawberries on the bottom of a small serving dish. Set aside. In a blender, combine millet, water, pineapple, salt and vanilla until consistency is like pudding. Add more water if necessary. Pour over strawberry slices. Sprinkle with nuts, raisins, or decorate with sliced strawberries, kiwi or fresh pineapple slices.
ONE SERVING

Variation: Add juice of 1/2 lemon, 1 TBS. lemon rind and 2 tsp. honey for lemon flavored pudding.

OATMEAL BREAKFAST MUFFINS
2.9 grams of fat per serving

1 1/4 cups rolled oats, uncooked
3/4 tsp. cinnamon
1/2 cup raisins
1/2 cup chopped dates
1/2 cup unsweetened crushed pineapple, drained
1 large apple, peeled, cored and chopped
1 egg white
1 1/2 tsp. Rumford aluminium free baking powder
1 tsp. vanilla extract
1/8 tsp. sea salt
vegetable cooking spray

Combine the oats, raisins, dates and cinnamon in large mixing bowl. Set aside. Combine remaining ingredients in container of electric blender, and process until smooth. Add pineapple mixture from blender to dry ingredients you set aside. Stir until well mixed. Spoon mixture evenly into muffin pan coated with vegetable cooking spray. Bake at 350 degrees for 35 minutes. These cakes will **not** rise during baking. (Yield 12 muffins) *ONE SERVING = 1 muffin*

Alternate: Make mini-muffins in a 24 muffin pan and freeze. Use for snacking, for breakfast or for brown-bag lunches.

ORANGE PANCAKES
2.6 grams of fat per serving

1 cup whole wheat flour
1 tsp. Rumford aluminum free baking powder
1/4 tsp. cinnamon
1 egg white
1/2 cup fresh squeezed orange juice
1/2 cup nonfat plain yogurt
1/2 tsp. canola oil
vegetable cooking spray

Combine the dry ingredients in a medium size mixing bowl. In a smaller bowl, beat the egg white and add orange juice, yogurt and oil. Add to the dry ingredients and stir until combined. Spoon batter onto a hot griddle or fry pan sprayed with vegetable cooking spray. Cook until golden brown on both sides. Serve with plain nonfat yogurt or unsweetened apple sauce. Yield 10-12 medium pancakes. *ONE SERVING = 3 pancakes*

OUTSTANDING OATS
6.3 grams of fat per serving

1/2 cup uncooked rolled oats (not instant)
1 TBS. unsulphured raisins or currants
6 raw, unsalted almonds
1 TBS. plain nonfat yogurt
1 apple, grated
distilled or spring water, boiling

Cover oats and raisins with boiling water. Soak 4-5 minutes. Add almonds, yogurt, and grated apple. Stir to mix and serve.
ONE SERVING

RAISIN BREAKFAST GRAIN
1.5 grams of fat per serving

3 cups water
1/2 cup uncooked brown rice
1/4 cup uncooked millet
1/2 unpeeled apple, chopped
2 TBS. raisins
1/4 tsp. cinnamon

Combine all ingredients in a medium saucepan and bring to a boil over moderate heat. Stir, reduce heat, and simmer with lid on for 25 to 30 minutes or until water is absorbed and rice, millet mixture is tender. Do not stir while cooking. Serve with a little fresh orange juice or nonfat plain yogurt as a topping. *ONE SERVING*

RAISINS AND SPICE OATS
1.8 grams of fat per serving

1 1/2 cups cold water
2/3 cup uncooked rolled oats (not instant)
3 TBS. raisins
1/2 tsp. cinnamon
1/8 tsp. cloves
pinch coriander
1 tsp. honey

Add oats, raisins and spices to cold water and bring to a boil over medium heat stirring constantly. Reduce heat and simmer, stirring constantly for about three to six minutes or until the mixture is thick and creamy. Remove from the heat. Cover, and let stand for 1-2 minutes for a thicker consistency. Stir in honey before serving if desired. *ONE SERVING*

RICE PUDDING

3.0 grams of fat per serving

1 cup hot, cooked brown rice
1/4 cup egg beaters
1/4 cup nonfat yogurt
2 TBS. raisins
1 TBS. crushed or sliced raw almonds
1/2 tsp. cinnamon
dash nutmeg
dash vanilla extract

Mix all ingredients in a large bowl until blended. Transfer to a baking dish and warm in a pre-heated 300 degree oven to blend flavors. Serve with a tablespoon of nonfat yogurt. *ONE SERVING*

(This dish keeps well for 24 hours. Rice pudding makes an excellent snack served cold and is a great lunchbox treat for school aged children).

SPANISH OMELET

13.1 grams of fat per serving

1/4 cup water
1/4 cup onions, chopped
1/4 cup celery, chopped
1/4 cup green pepper, chopped
1/4 cup zucchini or crookneck squash, chopped
2 TBS. water
1/2 cup tomato, chopped
2 whole eggs
1 tsp. butter
1/4 cup parsley, scissor-snipped

In a heavy skillet begin cooking onions in water over medium heat reducing heat to low when water begins to boil. Add celery, green pepper and squash and continue cooking until vegetables are soft. Do not overcook. Add tomatoes. Reduce heat to simmer. Cover pan. Beat eggs in a separate bowl. Melt butter in skillet with cooked vegetables over low heat. Pour eggs into pan and allow to cook gently. When done, fold in half to form omelet, remove from pan. Sprinkle with parsley and serve. *ONE SERVING*

ALTERNATE: **Use one cup of egg beaters to replace the whole eggs and reduce the fat grams to 4.5 per serving.**

VERY EASY FRENCH TOAST
2.2 grams of fat per serving

2 slices whole grain bread
1/2 cup egg beaters
1/4 cup nonfat milk
1/4 tsp. ground cinnamon
pinch of sea salt
1/16 tsp. vanilla extract
1/2 cup unsweetened applesauce
vegetable cooking spray

Cut bread diagonally into triangles. Place bread triangles on a cookie sheet. In a separate bowl combine egg beaters, milk, cinnamon, vanilla and salt with a hand blender or whisk. Pour over bread and allow to stand for 5 to 10 minutes turning once; bread will absorb liquid. Fry bread slices in a frying pan that is sprayed with vegetable cooking spray until browned and slightly crusty, turning once. Top with unsweetened apple sauce. *ONE SERVING*

SUGGESTION: **You may want to use 1 tsp. of butter to cook french toast. Add 5 grams of fat per serving.**

WEEKEND BREAKFAST QUICHE
6.0 grams of fat per serving

3/4 cup all purpose whole wheat flour
1/4 cup ground raw almonds
1/2 tsp. Rumford aluminum free baking powder
1/4 tsp. sea salt
1/3 cup skim milk
1 TBS. canola oil
1 cup egg beaters
1/2 cup chopped onion
1/2 cup chopped tomatoes
1/2 cup finely chopped broccoli florets
1/8 tsp. ground black pepper
1 TBS. chopped cilantro or parsley
vegetable cooking spray
fresh salsa if desired

Preheat oven to 400 degrees. Lightly spray a 9-inch pie pan or quiche dish with cooking spray. Set aside. In a medium-sized bowl, combine flour, ground almonds, baking powder and salt. Add milk and oil. Stir until just moistened. Lightly oil your fingers and remove dough from bowl. Pat dough out evenly onto the bottom and up the sides of the sprayed pan. Bake the dough in the oven for about 5-6 minutes, or until light brown. Remove from oven. Reduce oven temperature to 375 degrees. In another medium-sized bowl, combine remaining ingredients except cilantro (or parsley) and salsa. Pour egg mixture into baked crust. Bake for 25-30 minutes, or until center appears to be set. Remove from oven and let stand 5-10 minutes before serving. Sprinkle with cilantro or fresh parsley, and serve with salsa if desired. *FOUR SERVINGS*

THE MIDDAY MEAL

Your midday meal can be tasty, inexpensive, and easy to prepare whether eaten at home, in a restaurant, or from your lunchbox. Continue to experiment and you will add many of your own favorites to this list.

** Prepare a sandwich using a pita-pocket bread, whole grain bread or roll, or tortilla. Use lettuce, sliced tomatoes, sprouts, a small section of avocado, and mustard or ketchup to dress your sandwich. Try:

Turkey Breast	**Black Beans**
Chicken Breast	**Turkey Hot Dogs**
Turkey Bologna	**Grilled Chicken**
Canned Salmon	**Canned Tuna**
Vegetarian Sandwich	

** Use canned or homemade low-fat or fat free soups. Have a fresh tossed salad and a few crackers. Use lemon juice and safflower oil or packaged low-fat or nonfat salad dressing.

** Prepare any of the salads in the Salad Recipe section, or create one!

** Make an extra serving of any meal, refrigerate or freeze and serve at midday.

REMINDER: The best time to eat heavy protein is midday, because it takes approximately 8 hours to digest. Chicken, fish, turkey, or beef eaten late in the evening may keep you from sleeping well. Make sure your stomach is asleep before you are! **If you do eat heavy protein in the evening, please limit the number of times to 3-4 meals per week.**

EATING OUT
FAST FOOD RESTAURANTS

Fast food restaurants are beginning to revise their menus to offer a better selection of fat reduced foods. There are very few meals that we can honestly recommend because the fat grams are still so high. The following is a list of some of the lower fat items on their menus.

RESTAURANT NAME	GRAMS OF FAT
ARBY'S	
Junior Roast Beef Sandwich	9.0
Cheeseburger	5.0
BURGER KING	
Chicken Tenders (6 pieces)	10.0
Chef Salad	9.0
Chicken Salad	4.0
Garden Salad	5.0
Cheeseburger	15.0
Hamburger	12.0
CARL'S JR.	
Potatoes (Lite)	13.0
California Roast Beef	8.0
Charbroiler BBQ Chicken	5.0
Happy Star Hamburger	8.0
Soups	
Vegetable	3.0
Chicken noodle	1.0
CHICK-FIL-A	
Chicken Sandwich	8.9
Nuggets (8)	15.0
Chargrilled Chicken Sandwich	4.8
Chicken Garden Salad	2.0
Carrot and Raisin Salad	4.8
Chicken Soup	2.7

RESTAURANT NAME	GRAMS OF FAT
HARDEE'S	
Cheeseburger	14.0
Chicken Filet	16.0
Grilled Chicken Breast	9.0
Hamburger	13.0
Regular Roast Beef	9.0
Turkey Club	18.0
MCDONALD'S	
Chicken McNuggets	16.0
Hamburger	9.5
Cheeseburger	13.8
Salads	
Chef	13.0
Chicken	3.0
TACO BELL	
Bean Burrito	14.0
Chicken Burrito	10.0
Soft Chicken Taco	10.0
Pinto Beans	8.7
Taco	15.0
Tostada	11.0
WENDY'S	
Potatoes	
Chili Cheese	8.0
Chicken Breast	19.0
Grilled Chicken	11.0
1/4 lb. Hamburger	17.0
Chili (8 oz.)	8.0

TRADITIONAL RESTAURANTS

Restaurants are usually willing to prepare most meals according to your special requests. Simply ask the waitress or waiter to have the chef prepare your food with as little oil or butter as absolutely necessary. If a restaurant does not list what you want, ask for it. You will be surprised at how often you will hear, "Yes, we can do that!"

Choose traditional American style restaurants that feature fresh fish, grilled chicken or vegetarian dishes. Order steamed or stir-fry vegetables on the side, or you may prefer a salad with a baked potato or rice. Have a piece of bread or a roll, instead of dessert, unless they have a fat free or low-fat item.

ETHNIC RESTAURANTS

CHINESE RESTAURANTS
Order your dish without monosodium glutamate (MSG). MSG is a flavor enhancer which can cause severe headaches. Stir-fry chicken and vegetable dishes with steamed rice are excellent choices. Try Moo Shu Vegetables or Moo Shu Chicken which is served with a rice flour pancake and a sweet dark plum sauce.

ITALIAN OR PASTA
Pasta, a high complex carbohydrate is an excellent meal choice. Order with the marinara sauce. Have a salad with a little olive oil and fresh lemon juice as the dressing.

FISH HOUSES
Fish houses offer a wide variety of grilled and broiled fresh fish. Order a house salad and baked potato or rice.

PIZZA
The best selection is plain cheese pizza with about 11 grams of fat per slice. The more toppings, especially meats, the more fat. If you must have pizza, limit yourself to once a month.

MAIN DISHES

	GRAMS OF FAT	PAGE #
Apple-Chicken Stir-Fry	10.8	82
Barley Vegetable Chili	7.1	82
Black Bean Spaghetti	8.2	83
Chicken Pita-Pockets	9.9	84
Chicken Fried Rice	6.5	84
Dilled Salmon	10.2	85
Fried Cracked Wheat	13.9	86
Garden Rice Buffet	14.4	86
Grain Roast	2.0	87
Great 9 Bean Soup	less than one	88
Hearty Rice and Lentils	1.9	89
Laura's Lentil Stew	1.4	89
Orange Orange Roughy	10.1	90
Oven Crispy Chicken	4.6	90
Poached Red Snapper	5.0	91
Polynesian Fish	11.3	92
Roasted Turkey Dinner	12.0	92
Snapper Dijon	3.8	93
Saturday Nite Pasta	5.1	94
Spicy Chicken and Broccoli	7.4	95
Turkey Burger	9.3	95

APPLE-CHICKEN STIR-FRY

10.8 grams of fat per serving

1 TBS. sesame oil
2 boneless, skinless chicken breast halves, cut in thin strips
3 cups fresh broccoli florets
1 cup unpeeled cooking apple, cubed
1/4 cup celery, sliced thin
1 TBS. water
1/4 tsp. sea salt
1/8 tsp. curry powder
1/2 tsp. sesame seeds toasted

Heat oil in a large nonstick skillet; add chicken and stir-fry for about 3 minutes. Add broccoli, apple, celery, water, salt, and curry powder. Cover and simmer until vegetables are tender-crisp. Sprinkle with sesame seeds and serve hot. *TWO SERVINGS*

BARLEY VEGETABLE CHILI

7.1 grams of fat per serving

1 TBS. olive oil
2 cloves garlic, finely chopped
1/4 cup green pepper, chopped
1 TBS. chili powder (reduce for milder dish)
1/4 tsp. ground cumin
1 can plum tomatoes (28 ounces)
1 yellow squash, sliced into 1/2 inch-thick slices
1 can red kidney beans, drained and rinsed
1/3 cup pearled barley, cooked

Heat oil in large, nonstick saucepan. Add onion and garlic; saute 5 minutes. Stir in green pepper, chili powder, cumin, plum tomatoes and squash, breaking up tomatoes with spoon. Cover and simmer covered 15 minutes over medium-low heat. Add kidney beans and barley. Cover and cook for 5 minutes to heat. Top with nonfat plain yogurt and serve with green salad and steamed vegetables if desired. *TWO SERVINGS*

BLACK BEAN SPAGHETTI

8.2 grams of fat per serving

1 large yellow onion, sliced
1 red bell pepper, cut into strips
1 yellow bell pepper, cut into strips
2 TBS. olive oil
1 (16 oz.) can chopped whole tomatoes, undrained
1 (15 oz.) can black beans, drained and rinsed
1 (15 oz.) can red kidney beans, undrained
1 jar (3 1/2 oz.) capers, undrained
1/4 tsp. dried rosemary
1/4 tsp. dried basil
1/4 tsp. black pepper
3 cups cooked angel hair pasta
2 TBS. Parmesan cheese

Heat olive oil in a large skillet over medium-high heat. Add onion, and red and yellow peppers. Stir-fry until tender, stirring constantly. Add remaining ingredients and bring to a boil. Reduce heat and simmer for 30 minutes, stirring occasionally. Serve over cooked angel hair pasta, and sprinkle with Parmesan cheese.
FOUR SERVINGS

CHICKEN PITA-POCKETS
9.9 grams of fat per serving

1 clove garlic, finely chopped
1 medium yellow onion, chopped
1/4 cup fresh lime juice
2 tsp. olive oil
1/4 tsp. ground cumin
1/4 tsp. sea salt
1 TBS. chopped fresh cilantro
2 boneless, skinned chicken breast halves (4 ounces each),
cut into 1 inch-wide strips
1 sweet red pepper, cored, seeded and cut into thin strips
2 whole wheat pita-pocket breads

Combine garlic, lime juice, olive oil, cumin, salt, cilantro, and onion
in medium-size bowl. Add chicken and peppers. Cover and
marinade in the refrigerator for at least 30 minutes. Warm a large
nonstick skillet over medium-high heat. Saute the chicken and
vegetables in the marinade for 15 minutes or until chicken is done.
Place the chicken mixture in pita-pockets, dividing equally. Add
chopped lettuce, salsa and nonfat plain yogurt to the pita bread.
Serve with black beans if desired. *TWO SERVINGS*

CHICKEN FRIED RICE
6.5 grams of fat per serving

1 1/2 cups cooked brown rice
1/4 cup chopped green onion
1/4 cup egg beaters
1 carrot, thinly sliced and steamed until tender-crisp
1/2 cup green peas, frozen
1 cup cooked chicken, cubed (or turkey)
a pinch of garlic powder
1/2 cup mung bean sprouts
1 tsp. olive oil
reduced sodium soy sauce

Heat oil in deep skillet or wok. Pour egg into pan and scramble. When done, remove egg and set aside. Add onion and bean sprouts to pan. Cook for less than 1 minute. Remove from pan. Put the rice into the pan, add cooked egg, onion, sprouts, and all of the other ingredients. Mix and stir-fry till hot. Use a little water if necessary to keep the rice from sticking to the pan. Serve with a little soy sauce if desired. *TWO SERVINGS*

DILLED SALMON
10.2 grams of fat per serving

4 oz. salmon steak
1/2 tsp. butter, melted
1 TBS. lemon juice
1 tsp. dried dill
cayenne pepper, dash
vegetable cooking spray

Spray grill, skillet, broiler pan or baking dish with vegetable cooking spray. Brush fish with butter and lemon juice, sprinkle with dried dill. If baked, top fish with fresh dill sprigs. Try other herbs such as basil, tarragon, parsley, rosemary, chives. These steaks can be grilled, broiled, pan sauteed or baked. Cook about 10 minutes per inch of fish and turn after 5 minutes (except when baked).
ONE SERVING

"FRIED" CRACKED WHEAT
13.9 grams of fat per serving

1 cup cracked wheat
1 whole egg
1 egg white
4 tsp. sesame oil, divided in half
1 cup diced chicken, uncooked
1/2 cup broccoli, chopped
1/2 cup carrots, diced
1/4 cup green onions, sliced
1 clove garlic, minced
1/2 cup water chestnuts, chopped
1/2 cup frozen green peas, thawed
1/4 cup reduced sodium soy sauce
1/8 tsp. ground ginger

Place cracked wheat in a large mixing bowl; cover with water 2 inches above wheat. Soak for one hour and drain thoroughly. Combine egg and egg white in a small bowl and stir until blended. Heat 2 tsp. of the oil in a small skillet over medium heat, tilting the pan to coat the bottom. Pour in the egg mixture, and cook without stirring until the eggs begin to set. Carefully flip the eggs over and cook until done. Remove eggs from pan and let them cool. Cut eggs into thin (1/4 inch) strips. Set aside. Add remaining 2 teaspoons of oil to wok or large Dutch oven. Heat on medium heat. Add chicken, broccoli, carrots, green onions, and garlic. Stir-fry until chicken is done. Add cracked wheat, egg strips, water chestnuts, peas, soy sauce and ginger. Toss gently and serve. **TWO SERVINGS**

GARDEN RICE BUFFET
14.4 grams of fat per serving

1 tsp. olive oil
3/4 cups brown rice, cooked
1/2 small white onion, diced
2 cloves garlic, crushed
1 TBS. ginger root, grated fine
1/2 cup broccoli florets

1 carrot, sliced thin and diagonally
1/2 celery stalk, sliced thin and diagonally
1/4 cup snow pea pods
1/4 cup frozen green peas
4 oz. cooked turkey, cubed
vegetable cooking spray

Coat a large skillet with vegetable cooking spray, add olive oil and heat. Saute onions, garlic and ginger a few minutes. Beginning with the broccoli, saute vegetables being careful not to overcook Saute only long enough to warm them. Add green peas. The pea pods and turkey are added last to warm them. Vegetables should be slightly crisp. Stir in rice, and **gently** combine with vegetable turkey mixture. *ONE SERVING*

GRAIN ROAST

2.0 grams of fat per serving

1 1/2 cups cooked red beans (kidney or other variety)
3/4 cup rolled oats, uncooked
1 cup brown rice, cooked
6 nuts (chopped, <u>raw</u> almonds or walnuts)
1/4 cup egg beaters
1 cup Hunt's Tomato Sauce Special
1/8 tsp. each of sweet basil and thyme
1/4 tsp. sea salt
1/4 tsp. garlic powder
1 small onion, chopped
vegetable cooking spray

Mix all ingredients together in a large bowl slightly mashing beans. Press into a loaf pan sprayed with vegetable cooking spray. Bake 45 minutes to 1 hour at 350 degrees. Slice and serve.
FOUR SERVINGS

GREAT 9 BEAN SOUP
less than 1 gram of fat per serving

2 cups of 9 Bean Mix (see *NINE BEAN MIX* below)
2 quarts of de-fatted chicken broth
1 large onion, chopped
2 cloves garlic, minced
1 tsp. sea salt
2 cans of stewed tomatoes, Del Monte Original Recipe (No Salt)

Place 2 cups of the 9 Bean Mix in a Dutch oven or large pot. Cover with water 2 inches above beans. Soak overnight or for 24 hours for best results. Drain beans and return to Dutch oven or large pot. Add de-fatted chicken broth and rest of ingredients. Stir to mix. Cover and bring to a boil, reduce heat and simmer for 2 hours or until beans are tender. Stir occasionally. For a thicker soup, remove 1/4 of the soup, and blend in blender. Return to pot and stir to mix. *SIX SERVINGS*

HOW TO PREPARE 9 BEAN MIX:
Use 1 (dry) cup of <u>each</u> of the following:
black-eyed peas
black beans
red kidney beans
pinto beans
great northern beans
split peas
lentils
navy beans
barley pearls

HEARTY RICE AND LENTILS

1.1 grams of fat per serving

1/2 cup brown rice, uncooked
1/2 cup green lentils, uncooked
3 cups water, or de-fatted chicken broth
sea salt to taste
lemon juice to taste
curry powder to taste

Rinse rice and lentils in a strainer and add to water or broth in a covered pot. Bring to a boil. Reduce heat to low and cook covered until done, about 35-40 minutes. Do not stir contents or remove lid while cooking. When the liquid is absorbed, remove from heat and let set for 5-10 minutes. Fluff with a fork. Serve as a side dish or with vegetables for a main meal. Season with sea salt, lemon juice, and curry powder to taste. *TWO SERVINGS*

LAURA'S LENTIL STEW

1.4 grams of fat per serving

2 cups green lentils, uncooked
4 cups de-fatted chicken broth
4 cups water
1 large yellow onion, diced
2 stalks celery, sliced
2 cups fresh green beans, cut in 1-inch pieces
3 medium carrots, sliced
1 cup frozen corn
3 white potatoes, cubed
sea salt to taste

Soak lentils overnight in enough water to cover. Pour water off when ready to prepare dish. In a large pot or Dutch oven add drained lentils, broth, celery and onion. Bring to a boil, reduce heat and cook 1 hour. Add green beans, carrots, and corn, then cook another 1/2 hour. Then add cubed potatoes and cook another 1/2 hour or until potatoes are done. Season with sea salt to taste.
FOUR SERVINGS

ORANGE ORANGE ROUGHY
10.1 grams of fat per serving

1/3 cup fresh orange juice
1 orange roughy filet (about 4 ounces)
1 tsp. olive oil
1/2 TBS. dried tarragon
coarsely ground black pepper, pinch
grated rind of 1 orange

Preheat the oven to 325 degrees. Pour the orange juice into a shallow baking dish large enough to hold the fish. Brush the fish lightly with oil on both sides and place in baking dish. Combine the tarragon, pepper, and orange rind in a small bowl, and sprinkle over the fish, patting it lightly to form a thin crust. Bake until fish flakes easily when tested with a fork, 20 to 25 minutes. Using a long metal spatula carefully transfer the fish to a serving dish. (The fish may release a lot of liquid while cooking, just discard it.) Serve immediately. *ONE SERVING*

OVEN CRISPY CHICKEN
4.6 grams of fat per serving

1 chicken breast, half, boneless and skinless
2 TBS. egg beaters
1/2 cup Kellogg's Nutri-Grain Wheat Cereal, crushed
1/2 tsp. butter, melted
dash of sea salt
vegetable cooking spray

Wash and dry chicken with paper towel. Dip chicken in egg beaters and coat with crushed cereal. Place chicken into a baking pan sprayed with vegetable cooking spray. Drizzle melted butter on top of coated chicken. Bake at 350 degrees for 30-45 minutes or until done. Season with sea salt. *ONE SERVING*

POACHED RED SNAPPER
5.0 grams of fat per serving

4 oz. red snapper
1/8 tsp. white pepper
1/2 cup water
1 medium stalk celery, cut into long, thin strips
1 medium carrot, scraped and cut into long, thin strips
1/2 medium onion, chopped
Caper Sauce (recipe below)

Rinse fish with cold water and pat dry with a paper towel. Sprinkle with white pepper, and set aside. Pour 1/2 cup water into a 10-inch skillet. Heat water over medium heat until water starts to "quiver." (Do not boil) Add snapper and vegetables. Cover; reduce heat to low, and cook 8 minutes or until fish flakes easily when tested with a fork. (Do not allow water to boil.) Transfer fish and vegetables to a plate and spoon Caper Sauce over fish. Serve immediately.
ONE SERVING

CAPER SAUCE:
1/2 tsp. canola oil
1 TBS. water
2 tsp. fresh lemon juice
1 tsp. capers, drained
1/8 tsp. white pepper

Combine all ingredients in a small saucepan; stir until smooth. Cook over low heat stirring constantly for 3 minutes, or until sauce is thoroughly heated. Serve over cooked fish.

POLYNESIAN FISH
11.3 grams of fat per serving

4 oz. orange roughy filet
1 TBS. teriyaki sauce
1/2 tsp. safflower oil
1 green onion, chopped
1 tsp. fresh ginger root, minced
1/2 tsp. orange rind, grated
vegetable cooking spray

Rinse fish with cold water. Pat dry with a paper towel and place in a shallow baking dish. Combine teriyaki sauce, safflower oil, chopped onion, ginger root, and orange rind; mix well, and pour over fish. Turn fish in marinade to coat well. Cover and marinate in refrigerator at least 1 hour, turning fish occasionally. Spray rack of a broiler pan with vegetable cooking spray. Remove fish from marinade, discarding marinade. Place fish on rack, and broil 6 inches from heating element 5 minutes or until fish flakes easily when tested with a fork. Carefully transfer to a serving platter, and garnish with green onion if desired. *ONE SERVING*

ROASTED TURKEY DINNER
12 grams of fat per serving

One turkey breast - uncooked
1 stalk celery, sliced
1 carrot, sliced
1 cup brown rice, rinsed
4 cups de-fatted chicken broth
1/2 tsp. coriander
1/2 yellow onion, chopped
1 clove garlic, chopped
1/2 cup yellow squash, chopped
1/4 cup green bell pepper, chopped
1/2 cup zucchini, chopped
sea salt to taste

Take skin off turkey breast and place in roaster. Place garlic and all vegetables, brown rice, and chicken broth around turkey breast. Sprinkle coriander on the turkey. You may use any vegetables, such as broccoli, cauliflower, zucchini squash, or whatever you have on hand. Bake covered at 350 degrees for 1 1/2 hours or until rice is soft and turkey is tender. *ONE SERVING = 4 0Z.*

SNAPPER DIJON

3.8 grams of fat per serving

4 oz. red snapper
1/4 tsp. black pepper
1/2 tsp. ginger root, grated
1/8 cup Dijon mustard
1/2 TBS. fresh lemon juice
1/2 TBS. water
3/4 tsp. dried whole thyme
1/2 medium tomato, chopped

Cut one (15-inch) piece of heavy-duty aluminum foil . Rinse fish with cold water and pat dry with a paper towel. Place fish just off center of foil; sprinkle with pepper. In a separate bowl, combine mustard, water, thyme, ginger and tomato stirring well; pour evenly over fish. Seal foil securely and place on a baking sheet. Bake at 450 degrees for 10 minutes or until fish flakes easily when tested with a fork. Remove from foil, and serve. *ONE SERVING*

SATURDAY NITE PASTA
5.1 grams of fat per serving

2 cups green lentils, uncooked
6 cups water, spring or distilled
4 cloves garlic, crushed
1 large yellow onion, finely chopped
4 large carrots, finely diced
2 large celery stalks, finely chopped
1 large eggplant, cut into small cubes, skin left on
2 tsp. olive oil
5 oz. fresh spinach, washed and steamed
1 large can (28 oz.) crushed tomatoes
2 cups curly pasta, cooked, drained, and rinsed
1 1/4 tsp. Italian Seasoning
sea salt to taste
black pepper to taste
6 TBS. Parmesan cheese

Cook 2 cups of curly pasta according to package directions. Rinse and set aside. Cook 2 cups of lentils in 6 cups of boiling water. Reduce heat and simmer on low heat for 1 hour. Drain water reserving one cup for later. Set lentils aside. In a large Dutch oven or stew pot, heat oil and saute garlic, onions, celery, carrots and eggplant. Sprinkle Italian Seasoning over vegetables while sauteing. Do not overcook. The vegetables should be slightly crunchy. When vegetables are done, add tomatoes, lentils, spinach and pasta. Use the one cup reserved lentil cooking water to adjust the thickness to your taste. Allow to heat for 15-20 minutes, stirring occasionally. Add sea salt and pepper to taste. Sprinkle with Parmesan cheese before serving. *SIX SERVINGS*

Note: This is a wonderful tasting, very filling dish. It makes excellent leftovers and is certainly worth the effort to prepare. You may want to soak the lentils in water for 12-24 hours before cooking to reduce their musical quality.

SPICY CHICKEN AND BROCCOLI

7.4 grams of fat per serving

1 6 oz. chicken breast, cooked and cubed
1 tsp. olive oil
1 tsp. Mrs. Dash's Hot and Spicy seasoning
1 clove garlic, diced
1 cup broccoli florets
juice of 1 lime
reduced sodium soy sauce

Heat oil and saute garlic in heavy frying pan. Add Mrs. Dash seasoning and stir. Add broccoli and stir-fry until done. Add chicken to heat. Pour lime juice over finished dish. Use soy sauce to season when served. *ONE SERVING*

TURKEY BURGER

9.3 grams of fat per serving

4 oz. ground turkey
2 TBS. egg beaters
1/8 tsp. cumin
1/8 tsp. dry mustard
1/4 small onion, chopped
1 TBS. rolled oats, uncooked (optional)
dash sea salt

Mix all ingredients together. Shape into a patty and grill or broil. Serve on a whole grain bun with lettuce, tomato and mustard or ketchup if desired. *ONE SERVING*

SIDE DISHES

	GRAMS OF FAT	PAGE #
Baked Acorn Squash	less than one	98
Black Bean Medley	3.6	98
Cabbage and Green Beans	5.0	99
Carrot Rice Casserole	8.7	100
Cold Salmon Salad	8.0	100
Curried Wild Rice Salad	2.1	101
Dilled Asparagus	2.2	101
Easy Stir-Fry Squash	5.0	102
Green Beans with Shallots	5.0	102
Lemon Roasted Potatoes	7.5	103
Mexican Rice	1.8	103
Orange-Herb Rice	7.9	104
Pecan Sweet Potatoes	10.6	104
Pineapple Bulgar Wheat	4.2	105
Red Roasted Potatoes	9.2	105
Rice and Brussel Sprouts	7.0	106
Rio Grande Quinoa and Corn	4.6	106
Southern Red Rice	4.3	107
Spinach Balls	5.8	108
Squash and Onions	5.0	108
Steamed Garlic Broccoli	less than one	109
Stir-Fry Sesame Broccoli	7.0	109
Sunshine Medley	2.0	110
Two Cabbage Stir-Fry	5.0	111
Vermont Sweet Potatoes	less than one	111
Zucchini Tomato Bake	8.0	112

BAKED ACORN SQUASH WITH CURRANT SAUCE

less than one gram of fat per serving

1/2 baked acorn squash, seeds removed

CURRANT SAUCE:
1 TBS. currants or raisins
1/4 cup fresh orange juice
1/4 tsp. cinnamon
dash nutmeg
dash sea salt

In a blender, combine ingredients for currant sauce and blend on high speed until smooth. Heat on low in a small saucepan. Pour currant sauce into hot squash cavity and serve. *ONE SERVING*

BLACK BEAN MEDLEY

3.6 grams of fat per serving

1/2 tsp. olive oil
1/2 small onion, chopped
1 clove garlic, chopped
1 tsp. fresh cilantro, chopped (optional)
1/4 sweet green pepper, cored, seeded and chopped
1/2 can black beans, drained
1/2 cup frozen corn, thawed
1/4 tsp. sea salt
1/8 tsp. black pepper
1/4 tsp. ground cumin

Heat oil in nonstick skillet over medium-high heat. Add onion, garlic and green pepper; saute approximately 5 minutes. Add black beans, corn, salt, cumin, cilantro and pepper. Cook until heated through, about 5 minutes. Top with nonfat plain yogurt if desired. Serve with brown rice and a mixed green salad if desired. *ONE SERVING*

CABBAGE AND GREEN BEANS
5.0 grams of fat per serving

1 tsp. olive oil
3 TBS. de-fatted chicken broth
1/4 cup green cabbage, shredded
1/4 cup onion, chopped
1/8 tsp. sea salt or to taste
1/2 cup fresh green beans, cooked and drained, or 1/2 package frozen green beans, cooked and drained.

Heat oil and chicken broth in a skillet over medium heat. Add cabbage, onion, and salt. Saute for several minutes. Cover; reduce heat. Simmer for 15 minutes or until cabbage has cooked down to 1/2 the volume. (Cabbage may be refrigerated until serving time if desired). Add cooked green beans and heat for 5 minutes. Don't overcook the green beans - they should be bright green and still have a bit of crunch left. Overcooking also ruins cabbage, giving it a mushy texture and a strong taste. *ONE SERVING*

CARROT RICE CASSEROLE

8.7 grams of fat per serving

1 tsp. olive oil
6 large carrots, sliced
2 cups brown rice, cooked
1/3 cup finely chopped pecans
1 medium onion, finely chopped
1 carton soft tofu
3/4 cup nonfat milk
1/2 cup egg beaters
1/3 cup Parmesan cheese
sea salt to taste
pepper to taste
vegetable cooking spray

Steam carrots until barely tender; drain. Mix together cooked rice and pecans. In a small frying pan, saute onion in the olive oil. Set aside. In casserole sprayed with vegetable cooking spray, layer rice mixture, then onions, then carrots. Combine tofu, milk, egg beaters and cheese in a blender. Blend until smooth. Pour tofu mixture over layered casserole. Bake at 350 degrees for 30 minutes or until hot and bubbly. This is a good leftover dish which can be reheated. *SIX SERVINGS*

COLD SALMON SALAD

8.0 grams of fat per serving

1 large can red salmon
1 cup celery, diced
2 TBS. chopped dill pickle
1 TBS. chopped green pepper
1 tsp. chopped chives
1/3 cup nonfat plain yogurt
2 TBS. fresh lemon juice
assorted lettuce pieces
1 medium tomato, cut in wedges

Drain salmon, and mash with a fork until bones and skin are well blended. Add celery, pickle, green pepper, and chives to salmon;

mix well. In a separate bowl combine yogurt and lemon juice. Mix well and add to salmon. Mix well and chill for 2-3 hours. Serve with lettuce pieces and tomato wedges. *TWO SERVINGS*

CURRIED WILD RICE SALAD
2.1 grams of fat per serving

1 cup wild rice, cooked
1/4 cup carrot, grated
2 TBS. green pepper, finely chopped
2 TBS. green onions, sliced
3 large black olives, pitted, sliced
1 TBS. raisins
1 TBS. raw cashews, chopped
1/3 cup nonfat plain yogurt
3 TBS. unsweetened pineapple, undrained
2 tsp. lemon juice, fresh
1/4 tsp. curry powder

In a separate bowl combine yogurt, pineapple, lemon juice, and curry powder. Stir to mix. In another large bowl combine the rest of the ingredients. Add yogurt mixture to rice mixture. Stir until well blended. Chill and serve with salad greens if desired.
TWO SERVINGS

DILLED ASPARAGUS
2.2 grams of fat per serving

5-6 fresh asparagus spears cut into 1 inch pieces, steamed
1-2 tsp. dill weed
1/2 tsp. unsalted butter, melted
juice of 1/2 lemon
dash of sea salt

Mix all ingredients and pour over hot, steamed asparagus. Dill dressing is wonderful on all vegetables and fish.
ONE SERVING

EASY STIR-FRY SQUASH
5.0 grams of fat per serving

1 tsp. sesame oil
2 carrots, sliced thin
1 yellow or zucchini squash, sliced thin
1 small yellow onion, chopped
3 TBS. de-fatted chicken broth
1 tsp. reduced sodium soy sauce
1/2 cup egg beaters
2 tsp. dill weed

Heat oil and chicken broth in a skillet. Add soy sauce and
vegetables. Stir-fry till vegetables are tender. Add egg beaters and
dill weed. Mix until egg is scrambled into the vegetable mixture.
Serve hot. *ONE SERVING*

GREEN BEANS WITH SHALLOTS
5.0 grams of fat per serving

1 tsp. olive oil
1/4 lbs. fresh green beans, trimmed and cut in half
2 tsp. shallots, chopped (garlic or onions may be used)
1/4 cup water
2 TBS. de-fatted chicken broth

Heat oil and chicken broth in a heavy skillet or wok over medium
heat. Add green beans and shallots. Saute for about 2 minutes.
Add water and cover. Cook for 2 minutes longer, shaking skillet
occasionally. *ONE SERVING*

LEMON ROASTED POTATOES
7.5 grams of fat per serving

4 small red potatoes, washed and halved
1/8 cup fresh lemon juice
1 TBS. Parmesan cheese
1 tsp. olive oil
dash sea salt
dash black pepper
vegetable cooking spray

In a separate bowl mix ingredients and then add uncooked potatoes. Stir to coat. Arrange coated potatoes in an ovenproof baking dish sprayed with vegetable cooking spray. Roast in a 350 degree oven for 30-40 minutes or until potatoes are tender and crisp/brown. Turn potatoes 3-4 times during baking to baste. *ONE SERVING*

MEXICAN RICE
1.8 grams of fat per serving

1 large can Del Monte Original stewed tomatoes, unsalted
1/2 cup long grain brown rice, uncooked
3/4 cup water
1/2 to 1 tsp. chili powder

Mix all ingredients in saucepan, bring to a boil, reduce heat and cover. Simmer 30-40 minutes or until rice is tender and most liquid is absorbed. Season with sea salt and pepper to taste.
THREE SERVINGS

ORANGE-HERB RICE
7.9 grams of fat per serving

2 TBS. onion, chopped
2 TBS. butter, melted
2 cups water
1/2 tsp. orange rind, grated
1/2 cup fresh orange juice
1 tsp. sea salt
1/8 tsp. dried whole marjoram
1/8 tsp. thyme
1 cup long-grain brown rice, uncooked

Melt butter in a large saucepan. Saute onion until tender. Add water, orange rind, orange juice, salt, marjoram, and thyme; bring to a boil. Add rice and stir well. Cover and bring to a boil. Reduce heat and simmer 20 minutes or until rice is done. Let stand 5-10 minutes. Fluff with a fork and serve. *TWO SERVINGS*

PECAN SWEET POTATOES
10.6 grams of fat per serving

2 small, baked sweet potatoes, skin removed,
(or 1 1/2 cups water packed canned sweet potatoes; drained)
3/4 cup water packed crushed pineapple; drained
1/4 cup chopped pecans
1/2 cup egg beaters
vegetable cooking spray

Pre-heat oven to 350 degrees. In a medium-sized bowl, place sweet potatoes, egg beaters and drained pineapple. Blend ingredients with an electric mixer or a potato masher until ingredients are smooth. Place the mixture in a 2-quart baking dish sprayed with vegetable cooking spray. Smooth the top of the mixture with a spatula and spread the chopped pecans evenly over the top. Bake for 30 minutes. *TWO SERVINGS*

PINEAPPLE BULGAR WHEAT SALAD

4.2 grams of fat per serving

2 cups boiling water, spring or distilled
1 cup bulgar wheat, raw
1/2 tsp. sea salt
1 cup fresh (or frozen) pineapple, chunked
1/2 cup red bell pepper, chopped
2 inside stalks celery, chopped or
1/2 cup cucumber, chopped
3-4 scallions, thinly sliced
chopped chives
2 tsp. olive oil
3 TBS. lemon juice

Soak bulgar wheat in 2 cups boiling water until water is absorbed. Cool to room temperature, or refrigerate. Combine remaining ingredients. Stir in bulgar wheat last and serve. If you need to prepare salad early, leave out pineapple until the last moment.
TWO SERVINGS

RED ROASTED POTATOES

9.2 grams of fat per serving

4 small red potatoes, halved
6 cloves of garlic, separated but not peeled
2 tsp. olive oil
dash sea salt
dash pepper
vegetable cooking spray

In a separate bowl mix oil, salt, and pepper. Add halved potatoes and stir to coat with olive oil mixture. Arrange coated potatoes in an ovenproof baking dish sprayed with a light coat of vegetable cooking spray. Tuck the garlic cloves in among the potatoes. Bake at 350 degrees for 30-40 minutes, or until potatoes are tender. Garlic will be soft. Squeeze garlic from the peel, and serve with the potatoes. The garlic will have a nutty, sweet flavor. *ONE SERVING*

Rice And Brussel Sprouts

9.0 grams of fat per serving

1 tsp. olive oil
6 brussel sprouts, washed and trimmed
1 TBS. green onion, chopped
1 clove garlic, minced
3/4 cup brown rice, cooked
sea salt to taste
fresh lemon juice as desired
vegetable cooking spray

In a saucepan steam brussel sprouts for 12 minutes or until tender. Drain and coarsely chop. Spray a heavy saucepan or skillet with cooking spray and heat over low heat. Add oil, green onion and garlic. Saute until tender, but not brown. Add chopped brussel sprouts; mix well. Add rice and toss gently. Season with sea salt, and a little fresh lemon juice if desired. *ONE SERVING*

Rio Grande Quinoa And Corn

4.6 grams of fat per serving

1 1/2 cups water
3 TBS. lemon juice
1 TBS. olive oil
1 1/2 TBS. cilantro, minced
1 cup fresh or frozen corn
sea salt to taste

1/2 cup quinoa or rice
1/4 tsp. cumin seeds, toasted
1 cup black beans, cooked
1 medium tomato, diced
3 TBS. red onion, chopped
black pepper to taste

To make dressing, combine lemon juice, olive oil, cilantro, salt and pepper and set aside. Bring 1 1/2 cups water to boil in a small saucepan and add corn; reduce heat and simmer until corn is tender. Drain corn, reserving 1 cup of the cooking liquid. Return the one cup of the cooking liquid to the saucepan and bring to a boil. Add quinoa or brown rice and toasted cumin seeds; cover and simmer about 10 minutes (20-25 minutes for rice) or until liquid is absorbed. Remove quinoa from heat and set aside 5 minutes. Fluff quinoa with a fork and transfer to a salad bowl; cool slightly.

Add corn, black beans, tomato and onion to quinoa. Toss with
dressing and chill. Best when served cold. **FOUR SERVINGS**

SUGGESTION: Makes an excellent leftover salad, or use some crackers
or tortillas and serve as a "chunky dip"

SOUTHERN RED RICE

4.3 grams of fat per serving

1 large onion, chopped
1/2 cup celery, chopped
1/2 cup green pepper, chopped
1 cup long-grain brown rice, uncooked
1 (16 oz.) can chopped whole tomatoes, undrained
1 cup water; divided
1/2 tsp. sea salt
1/4 tsp. black pepper
1/4 tsp. red pepper
1/8 tsp. hot sauce
vegetable cooking spray

Saute celery, onion, and green pepper in 1/2 cup of water in a nonstick fry pan or skillet until tender. Stir in remaining ingredients.
Lightly spray a 1 1/2-quart baking dish with vegetable cooking
spray. Pour rice mixture into baking dish and cover. Bake at 350
degrees for 25 minutes, or until rice is tender. Stir once after 15
minutes. **TWO SERVINGS**

Spinach Balls
5.8 grams of fat per serving

2 ten ounce packages chopped spinach, thawed and squeezed
to remove excess water
1 cup cooked millet
1/3 cup Parmesan cheese
2 TBS. melted butter
1/4 cup egg beaters
3/4 tsp. garlic salt
vegetable cooking spray

Mix all ingredients together in a large bowl. Make certain that the
spinach is well mixed with the grain. You can use a potato masher,
or a hand blender. Form into cocktail sized balls. Spray a cookie
sheet with vegetable cooking spray and place balls on the pan.
Bake at 350 degrees for 15-20 minutes or until the tops are brown
and the balls sizzle. Stick a colored toothpick into each spinach ball
after cooking for easy eating and decoration. *SIX SERVINGS*

ALTERNATE: The mixture can be made into bars similar in size to
brownies using an 8 x 8 glass baking dish

Squash And Onions
5.0 grams of fat per serving

1 tsp. olive oil
2 yellow squash, cut into 2-inch pieces
1 medium yellow onion, sliced in strips
1/4 tsp. oregano
1/4 cup water
sea salt to taste
1/2 tsp. reduced salt soy sauce

Heat the oil and soy sauce in a 2-quart saucepan, add the onions
and saute until transparent. Add the squash and oregano and
saute for another 2 or 3 minutes. Add the water and salt if desired.
Squash should be crisp. Do not overcook. *ONE SERVING*

STIR-FRIED SESAME BROCCOLI

7.0 grams of fat per serving

1 tsp. sesame oil
1/4 bunch broccoli
1/2 tsp. garlic, finely chopped
1/4 cup sliced water chestnuts (canned, drained)
1 tsp. toasted sesame seeds
1 TBS. reduced salt soy sauce

Separate broccoli into florets; peel and thinly slice the stems. Heat a wok or heavy skillet over medium heat. Add oil, soy sauce and garlic. Stir-fry for 30 seconds. Add broccoli stems. Stir-fry for 4 to 5 minutes or until tender-crisp. Add broccoli florets and the water chestnuts; cover. Steam for 3 to 4 minutes or until broccoli is tender-crisp, stirring occasionally. Sprinkle with toasted sesame seeds and serve. *ONE SERVING*

STEAMED GARLIC BROCCOLI

less than one gram of fat per serving

1/4 bunch broccoli
1 clove garlic, minced
1/2 cup water
sea salt to taste

Wash and chop the broccoli, separating the stems and florets. Place the broccoli stems in a 1 1/2-quart saucepan with the water and garlic; cover and steam for 4 minutes. Uncover and stir the stems; arrange the florets on top, then cover and steam for another 4 minutes. Use sea salt to taste. *ONE SERVING*

SUNSHINE MEDLEY
2.0 grams of fat per serving

1 cup raw sweet potatoes, cubed
1 cup carrots, sliced
1/2 cup yellow squash, sliced
1 small onion, quartered
1 TBS. dill weed
1/2 cup fresh lemon juice
1 tsp. honey
1/2 tsp. sea salt
1 cup cooked pasta shells
1 TBS. Parmesan cheese

Steam the potatoes, carrots, and onion in a 2-quart pan using a stainless steel vegetable steamer (if you have one) until the potatoes and carrots are nearly tender. Add the squash and continue steaming until the vegetables are tender. In a separate bowl combine the remaining ingredients. Toss the steamed vegetables in the sauce until well coated. Serve over cooked pasta shells, and sprinkle with Parmesan cheese. *TWO SERVINGS*

TWO CABBAGE STIR-FRY
5.0 grams of fat per serving

1 tsp. olive oil
1 TBS. hot water
1 tsp. cornstarch
1 small onion, chopped
1 tsp. fresh ginger root, chopped
1 cup red cabbage, thinly sliced
1 cup green cabbage, thinly sliced
1 TBS. reduced sodium soy sauce

Heat oil and soy sauce over medium heat in a wok or heavy skillet. Add onion and ginger root. Stir-fry for 1 minute. Add red and green cabbage. Stir-fry for 3 to 5 minutes or until cabbage is tender. In a small dish combine hot water and cornstarch. Mix well and add to vegetables. Bring to a boil, stirring constantly. Serve hot.
TWO SERVINGS

VERMONT SWEET POTATOES
less than one gram of fat per serving

1 large sweet potato, washed and scrubbed
1/4 tsp. cinnamon
1/8 tsp. maple flavoring
1/16 tsp. rum extract
2 TBS. hot water

Place washed sweet potato into a pot of boiling water. Cover and boil potato until tender. Drain and cool potato. Peel and mash it in a separate bowl. Add the cinnamon, maple flavoring, rum extract and hot water to the mashed potato. Beat until fluffy and serve.
ONE SERVING

ZUCCHINI TOMATO BAKE
8 grams of fat per serving

3 medium sized zucchini, sliced thin
1 small onion, sliced thin
1 TBS. olive oil
2 TBS. fresh chopped parsley
1 ripe tomato, sliced
sea salt to taste
black pepper to taste
1 tsp. Parmesan cheese
vegetable cooking spray

Steam zucchini and set aside. In a heavy skillet, saute onion in olive oil until tender and then add chopped parsley. Remove from heat. Spray a 1-quart baking dish with vegetable spray. Put a layer of drained zucchini in dish, then a layer of sliced tomatoes, then onion mixture. Sprinkle with sea salt and pepper to taste. Sprinkle Parmesan cheese on top. Bake at 350 degrees for 30 minutes.
ONE SERVING

CHAPTER ELEVEN

EXERCISE THE MUSCLES THAT BURN FAT

"There is no exercise better for the heart
than reaching down and lifting people up."
John Andrew Holmes

We all need to exercise, but exercise will not burn as many calories as the thermogenic effect of food.[1-4] What we eat affects our metabolism more than how much we exercise. Weight loss programs put too much emphasis on exercise as a primary way to burn calories. Many people find out after several months of exhausting workouts in classes, gyms, or in front of their television set, that very little weight, if any, is lost! In fact, a person can actually gain weight since exercising builds muscle and muscle weighs 2.5 times more than fat! **The "right" type of exercise can change the body's chemistry, not just burn a few calories.** Exhausting aerobic workouts are not necessary. The real advantage of adding exercise to the Genesis Way of life is not because one loses weight, but because the right kind of exercise will make the body a more efficient fat-burning furnace. The number of calories burned during the exercise period is not nearly as important as choosing an exercise that will work the muscle groups which fire up our metabolism long after the exercise is over! **The purpose of exercise is to increase our metabolism even when we are not exercising!**

Changing Attitudes About Exercise
Adding exercise to a low calorie diet does not increase weight loss potential. In fact, dieters who exercise lose no more weight than dieters who do not exercise says researcher Stephen Phinney of the Metabolic Unit of the University of Vermont Clinical Research Center.[5] Calorie-deficient diets destroy lean muscle and are not advantageous for building a fat-burning furnace. According to C. Wayne Callaway of the George Washington School of Medicine's Center for Clinical Nutrition, if a person undereats and exercises a lot, their metabolic rate can actually decrease.[5]

A few years ago the old saying "no pain, no gain," was the prevailing attitude when it came to exercising. Most people believed that if they wanted to burn fat, they had to exercise intensely. Experts are now realizing that longer periods of moderate exercise, rather than short periods of intense exercise, are more efficient in burning fat! When we exercise we want to burn fat, not just calories. New information about exercising suggest that different exercises require different durations in order to burn fat. At the beginning of any exercise, the calories burned are mostly glucose or sugar calories, not fat. When the muscles burn their glycogen reserves, then they begin to burn stored fat. For example, at the beginning of a walk, we burn ten percent (10%) fat and ninety percent (90%) sugar. After forty minutes of walking, we are now burning ninety percent (90%) fat and ten percent (10%) sugar. On the other hand, after only l5 minutes of jogging, the jogger is burning mostly fat.[6] Swimming, a good aerobic exercise, burns little fat no matter how long the exercise period. Our body "holds on" to the fat in order to keep warm and stay buoyant. Experts once believed that any exercise would help us burn fat, but again this has changed. The exercise we choose can actually be rated according to its **fat burning potential (FBP).**[6] Some examples are as follows:

Fat Burning Potential

1. Walking   - low, unless continued for 40 minutes or more
2. Jogging   - high, especially after 15 minutes
3. Cycling   - moderate, unless for 40 minutes or more
4. Swimming - low
5. Rowing   - high, uses large muscle groups
6. Stair-climb - high, especially after 15 minutes
7. Treadmill   - moderate to high, depending on incline and speed

Since fat is burned in the muscle, the best exercises to do are the ones that use large muscle groups rather than small ones. Exercising over a long time period increases the percentage of fat calories burned.

The S-Factors - The Three Classifications of Exercise

1. Stamina Exercise - These are the basic cardiovascular (heart, lung, and circulation) exercises like walking, running, calisthenics and aerobic fitness. If we use large muscle groups during a long time period, the muscles will burn some bodyfat. However, stamina exercise is primarily for the heart and lungs.

2. Stretching Exercise - These exercises do not burn fat, but they are an essential part of any exercise program. Stretching exercises help prevent injuries, improve flexibility, and reduce tension, back pain, and stiffness. Stretching helps keep muscles long, flexible and unknotted. Stretching exercises feel great!

3. Strength Exercise - These exercises work specific muscle groups by using small weights, free weights, weight machines or some other form of resistance equipment. Strength exercises focus exclusively on building and maintaining muscle mass.

Strength Training for Higher Metabolism

Muscle accounts for ninety percent (90%) of tissue metabolism.[6] For every 100 calories we eat, 90 calories should be burned in your muscles. However, if you lose muscle mass, either by frequent dieting, having a high percentage of bodyfat or just in the process of aging, you lose **metabolizing power!** Did you know that an infant is mostly muscle and water? As we age, the percent of muscle mass decreases and the percent of bodyfat increases. Calories not burned in the muscle are likely to be stored in the fat! People often say, "I can't eat the way I used to!"

Strength Training Superior to Aerobics for Muscle Mass
Many weight loss programs advocate calorie restriction and some form of exercise to help burn fat. Aerobic exercise such as walking, jogging and dancing is often the exercise of choice for most of these weight loss programs. However, Dr. Kenneth Cooper, whose first book, Aerobics, helped launch the exercise industry, has recently been quoted as saying that "lower body exercisers lose upper body muscle mass as they age." Cooper now says that aerobic exercise (stamina exercise) is "merely the foundation" for a

program. He believes that strength training is also important for muscle development. Dr. Bryant Stamford, professor of Allied Health at the University of Louisville, in Kentucky, sums up the the basic difference between strength training and stamina exercise in this way, "Weight training is like a salary, and aerobics is like a bonus." The benefits of stamina exercise (aerobics) end shortly after the exercise is over, whereas **strength training keeps the fat-burning furnace going long after the workout is over because it focuses on the primary metabolic tissue - muscle!**

Recently, studies were completed at the Exercise Physiology and Nutrition Laboratory at the University of Massachusetts Medical School [7] dealing with changes in bodyfat and muscle mass of dieters who were divided into 4 groups:

> 1. Nonexercisers
> 2. Aerobic exercisers
> 3. Strength trainers
> 4. Exercisers doing both aerobics and strength training

The following results confirm the superiority of strength training over aerobics for building more muscle mass. **The increased muscle mass means increased metabolizing power!**

> 1. Nonexercisers lost 9 pounds, but 11% of that was muscle! Calorie restricted diets destroy muscle!
> 2. Aerobic exercisers lost 10 pounds, but 1% of the weight lost was muscle! Aerobic exercise prevented the loss of muscle during dieting periods, but did not add any new muscle mass.
> 3. Strength trainers lost 9 pounds and **added 9%** new muscle mass to their bodies! Strength exercises **increase** the percent of metabolizing muscle tissue.
> 4. Exercisers doing both aerobics and strength training lost 13 pounds and added 4% new muscle mass to their bodies. Combining aerobic workouts with strength training increased weight loss. However, it was not as effective as strength training alone at building muscle mass.

All of the participants in these studies lost weight, but only the strength trainers increased lean muscle while losing bodyfat.

116

Remember, ninety percent (90%) of your metabolism takes place in the muscle. Muscle is metabolically active, fat is not! **Strength training is the perfect exercise because it replaces fat with muscle.** To make your body into an efficient fat-burning furnace you must increase your muscle mass and decrease bodyfat.

The Genesis Way 20-Minute Strength Training Workout

The Genesis Way recommends the following 20 minute strength training workout as the most efficient way to build muscle for **more metabolizing power**. We also recommend stretching and stamina exercises for a complete workout. However, if you can only spare 20 minutes a day, then **The Genesis Way 20-Minute Strength Training Workout is the best choice to help your body become a fat-burning furnace!**

Women should start with dumbbells that weigh about four to five pounds <u>each</u> and gradually, over a number of weeks, work up to ten pounds for each dumbbell. Men should begin with approximately ten pounds of weight for each dumbbell and gradually work up to twenty pounds for each dumbbell. Dumbbells can be purchased at sports shops or discount stores very inexpensively. Remember fat just sits there and does nothing! Muscle, on the other hand, is active tissue that burns fat! The more muscle tissue we have, the faster we burn fat. This workout is designed to work the biceps, triceps, chest, shoulders, abdominals, back, thighs, buttocks, and calves.

We are not interested in becoming a muscle bound Arnold Schwartznager. We are lifting light weights in order to work the different muscle groups, without building big muscles. The key to the success of The Genesis Way 20-Minute Strength Training Workout is repetitions. Begin with a comfortable set of ten or twelve repetitions for each exercise and as the body gets in better shape, increase the sets to three sets of twelve repetitions for each exercise. Do these strength training exercises every other day and alternate with an aerobic exercise like walking on the other days.

Upper Body Workout

Alternate Dumbbell Curl - Stand with feet slightly a part, holding a dumbbell in each hand. Palms should be facing up and arms hanging at your sides. Starting with the left arm bend your arm until it reaches your shoulder. Slowly return the left arm to your side again, remembering to keep your arm close to your side. Repeat the same motion with the right arm and when you finish each arm once, that is one repetition. **Develops and shapes entire bicep muscle or upper arm area.**

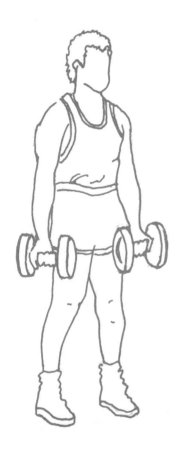 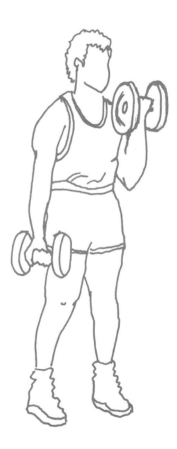

Perfect Sitting Curl - Sit in a chair and hold a dumbbell in your right hand with palm up, arm extended toward the floor. Bend over and position your left elbow on your left inner knee. Curl your left arm until the dumbbell reaches chin level and slowly return to beginning position. Repeat ten or twelve times with the right arm only. Change arms and repeat the exercise with your left arm. **Develops and shapes the bicep muscle or upper arm area.**

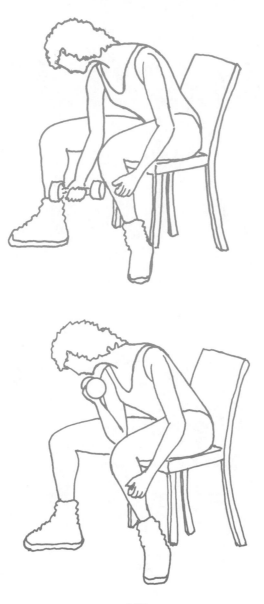

One-Arm Tricep Extention - Standing with feet slightly apart, bend at the waist. Holding a dumbbell in your right hand, palm toward body, arm at your side, curl up to a right angle. As you straighten your right arm, extend it back as far as possible. After doing ten or twelve repetitions, change to the left arm and repeat exercise. **Shapes the entire tricep muscle or underarm.**

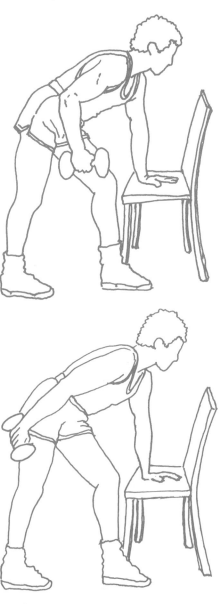

One-Arm Overhead Tricep Extention - Sit in a chair, with dumbbell in right hand and palm facing toward the body. Raise dumbbell over your head with arm extended. Keeping right arm close to your head, lower the dumbbell behind your head and then return to the starting position. After ten or twelve repetitions, switch to the left arm. **Tightens tricep muscle or underarm area.**

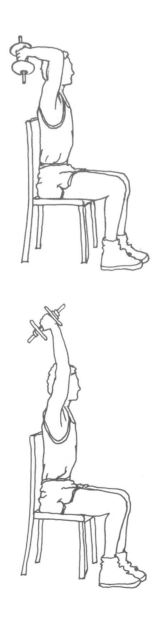

Dumbbell Flye - Lie on a flat exercise bench with arms holding dumbbells fully extended above your chest (dumbbells touching). Extend your arms outward and downward in an arcing motion. Return to starting position and repeat ten to twelve repetitions. **Shapes the entire chest region.**

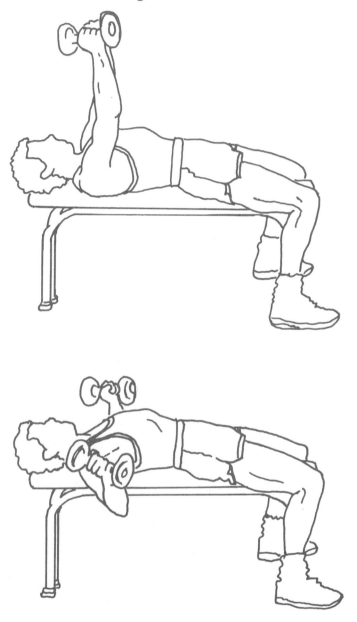

Standing Side Lateral - With feet slightly apart and holding a dumbbell in each hand, touch dumbbells in front of you about waist level. Extend your arms upward and outward until the dumbbells reach neck height and then return to starting position in front of you. Repeat ten to twelve times. **Shapes the entire deltoid muscle or shoulder.**

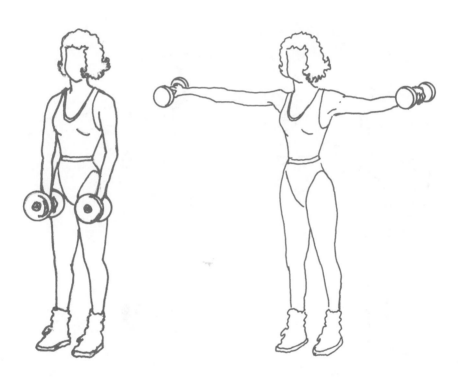

Bent Lateral - Sit in a chair or stand with feet slightly apart holding a dumbbell in each hand. Bend at the waist and touch dumbbells. Extend your arms outward until they are parallel with the floor. Return to starting position and repeat exercise ten or twelve repetitions. **Develops the deltoid muscle or shoulder.**

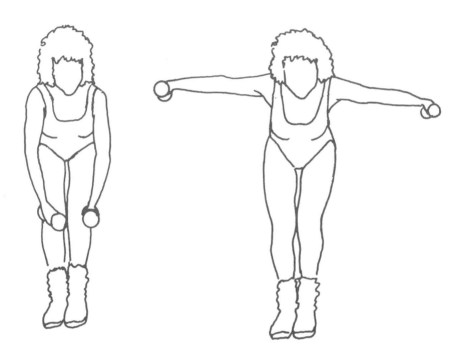

Lower Body Workout

Normal Squat - Stand with feet about eight inches apart, holding the dumbbell in each hand. Dumbbells should be at your sides with palms facing in and back straight. Standing on the "balls" of your feet, descend to the point where the buttocks touch the chair positioned behind you. Then return to standing position. Repeat ten or twelve repetitions. **Shapes the quadricep muscle or front thigh.**

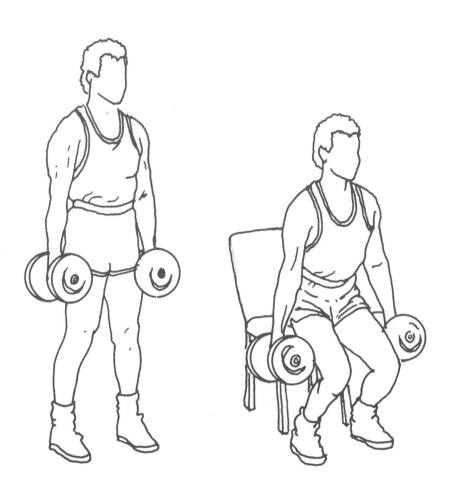

Lunge - Stand with feet six to eight inches apart holding a dumbbell in each hand (palms facing in). With back straight and dumbbells down at your sides, step forward about two and a half feet with the left leg bending at the knee (lunging motion). Return to start position and repeat with the left leg until you have completed ten to twelve repetitions. Without resting, repeat with the other leg. **The lunge is excellent for the quadriceps muscle or front thigh.**

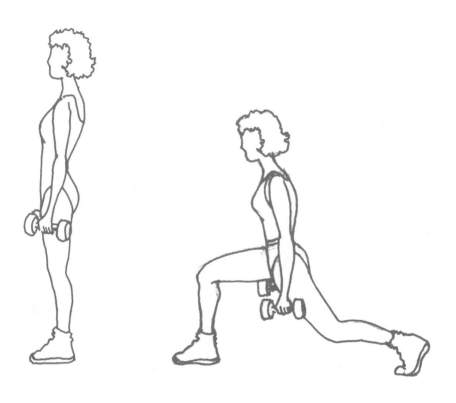

Standing Calf Raise - Stand with left foot on a two to four inch piece of wood so that the heel is resting on the floor. Hold the back of a chair with your right hand while holding a dumbbell at your side with the left hand. Bend the right leg and raise it off the floor. Lift left heel off the floor and raise onto your left toes. Repeat the movement until ten or twelve repetitions are completed. Repeat exercise with the right foot. **Shapes the calf muscle.**

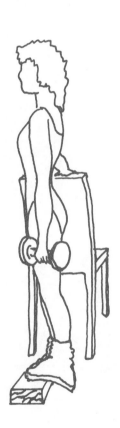
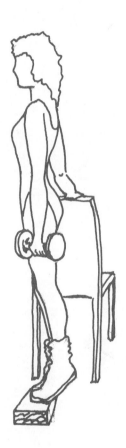

Crunches - Lie down on the floor with your legs bent at a right angle and the lower half of the legs resting on a chair. Tuck the chin to the chest and rest the arms in a criss-cross position on the chest. Curl the body until the shoulders are completely off the floor. Return to the floor again and do as many as possible. A variation on the straight crunch is to cross the right shoulder to the left side. After several repetitions, repeat with the other shoulder. **Tightens and tones the entire upper abdominal area or the stomach.**

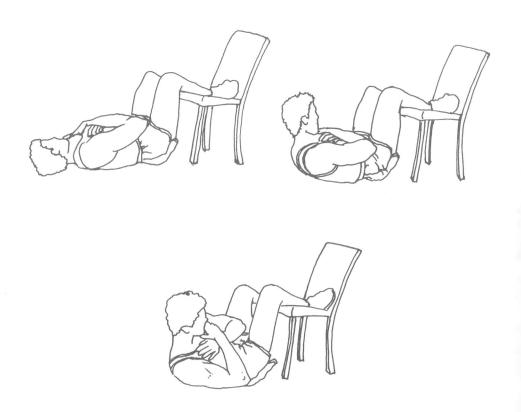

In the beginning, **The Genesis Way 20-Minute Strength Training Workout** may take you a little longer to complete. Concentrate on each muscle that you are working and take your time, being very deliberate with each exercise. These simple, yet effective exercises can do more for your metabolism than an hour of aerobics! You are building lean muscle and that means more **metabolizing power!**

BEGIN, THE REST IS EASY

The Genesis Way of life will help you achieve your desired fat loss, without restricting calories or forcing you to feel "starved." You can break the fat barrier the Genesis Way! As you begin your new lifestyle you will:

1. Develop a healthy way of eating
2. Eat less of the foods that easily store as fat
3. Eat more thermogenic foods
4. Reduce your percentage of bodyfat while increasing lean muscle
5. Boost your metabolism to burn calories
6. Increase your energy level
7. Feel healthier and more alive

The Genesis Way is a healthy way of life not only for you, but for your family, friends, and co-workers. As you become leaner and healthier, everyone will ask you how you did it! And you will be able to say with confidence,

"There's only one way...The Genesis Way!

REFERENCES

Introduction

1. Lissner, L., Odell, P.M., D'Agostino, R.B., et al. "Variability of Body Weight and Health Outcomes in the Framingham Population." The New England Journal of Medicine (June 27, 1991); Vol. 324, no. 26: 1839-1844.

2. Blackburn, G.L., Wilson, G.T., Kanders, B.S., et al. "Weight cycling: the experience of human dieters." The American Journal of Clinical Nutrition (1989); 49:1105-9.

Chapter One

1. Dreon, D.M., Frey-Hewitt, B., Ellsworth, N., et al. "Dietary fat: carbohydrate ratio and obesity in middle-aged men." The American Journal of Clinical Nutrition (1988); 47:995-1000.

2. Masoro, E.J. "Biochemical mechanisms related to the homeostatic regulation of lipogenesis in animals." Journal of Lipid Research. (1962); Vol. 3, no. 2:149-164.

3. Blackburn, G.L., Wilson, G.T., Kanders, B.S., et al. "Weight cycling: the experience of human dieters." The American Journal of Clinical Nutrition (1989); 49:1105-9.

4. Braitman, L.E. "Obesity and caloric intake: The National Health and Nutrition Examination Survey of 1971-1975." (HANES I). The Journal of Chronic Disease (1985) Vol. 38, no. 9:727-732.

5. Tremblay, A., Despres, J.P., Maheux, J. " Normalization of the metabolic profile in obese women by exercise and a low fat diet." Medicine and Science in Sports and Exercise. (1991); Vol. 23, 12:1326-1331.

6. Sheppard, L., Kristal, A.R., Kushi, L.H. "Weight loss in women participating in a randomized trial of low-fat diets." American Journal of clinical Nutrition. (1991); 54:821-828.

7. Thomas, C.D., Peters, J.C., Reed, G.W., et al. "Nutrient balance and energy expenditure during ad libitum feeding of high-fat and high-carbohydrate diets in humans." American Journal of Clinical Nutrition. (1992); 55:934-942.

8. Sims, E.A. "Expenditure and storage of energy in man." Journal of Clinical Investigation. (April 1987); 79:1019-1025.

9. Wood, J.D., Reid, J.T. "The influence of dietary fat on fat metabolism and body fat deposition in meal-feeding and nibbling rats." British Journal of Nutrition. (1975); 34:15-24.

10.   Dreon, D.M., Frey-Hewitt, B., Ellsworth, N., et al. "Dietary fat: carbohydrate ratio and obesity in middle-aged men." American Journal of Clinical Nutrition (1988); 47:995-1000.

11.   Jones, R. "Role of Dietary Fat in Health." Journal of the American Oil Chemists' Society." 51:251-254.

12.   Berry, E.M., Hirsch, J., Most, J., et al. "The role of Dietary Fat in Human Obesity." International Journal of Obesity. (1986); 10:123-131.

13.   DeHaven, J., Sherwin, R., Hendler, R., et al. "Nitrogen and Sodium balance and sympathetic-nervous-system activity in obese subjects treated with a low-calorie protein or mixed diet." the New England Journal of Medicine. (February 28, 1980); vol. 302, no. 9: 477-482.

14.   Felig, P. "Editorial Retrospective. Very-low-calorie protein diets." The New England Journal of Medicine. (March 1, 1984); vol. 310, 9:589-591.

15.   Jung, R.T., Shetty, P.S., Barrand, M., et al. "Role of catecholamines in hypotensive response to dieting." British Medical Journal. (1979); 1:12-13.

16.   Nilsson, L.H., Hultman, E. "Liver Glycogen in Man - the Effect of Total Starvation or a Carbohydrate-Poor Diet Followed by Carbohydrate Refeeding." Scandinavian Journal of Clinical Laboratory Investigation. (1972); 32:325-330.

17. Liddle, R.A., Goldstein, R.B., Saxton, J. "Gallstone Formation During Weight-Reductioln Dieting." Archives of Internal Medicine. (1989); 149:1750-1753.

18. Brownell, K., Greenwood, MRC., Stellar, E., et al. "The effects of repeated cycles of weight loss and regain in rats." Physiology of Behavior. (1986); 38:459-64.

19. Bessard, T., Schutz, Y., Jequier, E., "Energy Expenditure and Postprandial Thermogenesis in Obese Women Before and After Weightloss." The American Journal of Clinical Nutrition 38. (November 1983); 680-693.

20. Blackburn, G.L., Wilson, G.T., Kanders, B.S., et al. "Weight cycling: the experience of human dieters." The American Journal of Clinical Nutrition (1989); 49:1105-9.

21. Lissner, L., Odell, P.M., D'Agostino, R.B., et al. "Variability of Body Weight and Health Outcomes in the Framingham Population." The New England Journal of Medicine (June 27, 1991); Vol. 324, no. 26:1839-1844.

22. Reed, D.R., Conrera, R.J., Maggio, C., et al. "Weight cycling in female rats increases dietary fat selection and adiposity." Physiology of Behavior. (1988); 42:389-95.

23. Lincoln, A., Food for Athletes, Contemporary Books Inc., 1979, 292 pages, reference page 106.

Chapter Two

1. U.S. Department of Agriculture and U.S. Department of Health and Human Services, 1980, "Nutrition and Your Health- Dietary Guidelines for Americans.", Washington, D.C., pages 1-20.

2. Flatt, J.P., Ravussin, E., Acheson, K.J., et al. "Effects of Dietary Fat on Postprandial Substrate Oxidation and on Carbohydrate and Fat Balances." Journal of Clinical Investigation (September 1985); 76:1019-1024.

3. Roberts, L., "Diet and Health in China," Science (1988); 240:27.

4. Sheppard, L., Kristal, A.R., Kushi, L.H., "Weight loss in women participating in a randomized trial of low-fat diets." American Journal of Clinical Nutrition (1991); 54:821-8.

5. Braitman, L.E. "Obesity and caloric intake: The National Health and Nutrition Examination Survey of 1971-1975." (HANES I). The Journal of Chronic Disease. (1985) Vol. 38, no. 9:727-732.

6. Krombout, D., "Changes in energy and macronutrients intake in 871 middle age men during 10 years of follow-up, (Zutphen Study)." American Journal of Clinical Nutrition, (1983); 37:287-294.

7. Dreon, D.M., Frey-Hewitt, B., Ellsworth, N., et al. "Dietary fat: carbohydrate ratio and obesity in middle-aged men." American Journal of Clinical Nutrition (1988); 47:995-1000.

8. Blaza, S., Garrow, J.S. "Thermogenic response to temperature, exercise and food stimuli in lean and obese women, studied by 24 h direct calorimetry." British Journal of Nutrition. (1983); 49:171-180

9. Romieu, I., Willett, W.C., Stampfer, M.J., et al. "Energy intake and other determinants of relative weight." American Journal of Clinical Nutrition. (1988); 47:406-12.

10. Schlundt, D.G., Taylor, D., Hill, J. D., Sbrocco, T., Pope-Cordell, J., Kassen, T., Arnold, D. "A behavioral taxonomy of obese female participants in a weight loss program." American Journal of Clinical Nutrition. (1991); Vol. 53. 1151-1158.

11. Masoro, E.J. "Biochemical mechanisms related to the homeostatic regulation of lipogenesis in animals." Journal of Lipid Research. (1962); Vol. 3, no. 2:149-164.

12. Acheson, K.J., Schultz, Y., Bessard, E., et al. "Nutritional influences on lipogenesis and thermogenesis after a carbohydrate meal." American Journal of Physiology. (January 1984); 246(1 PT 1)E62-70.

13. D'Alessio, D.A., Kavle, E.C., Mozzoli, M.A., et al. "Thermic Effect of Food in Lean and Obese Men." Journal of Clinical Investigation. (1988); Vol. 81. 1781-1789.

14. Bessard, T., Schultz, Y., Jequier, E. "Energy expenditure and postprandial thermogenesis in obese women before and after weight loss." the American Journal of clinical Nutrition. (November 1983); 38:680-693.

15. Blackburn, G.L., Wilson, G.T., Kanders, B.S., et al. "Weight cycling: the experience of human dieters." The American Journal of Clinical Nutrition (1989); 49:1105-9.

16. Miller, D.S., Mumford, P., Stock, M.J. " Gluttony. Thermogensis in Overeating Man." American Journal of Clinical Nutrition. (November 1967); Vol. 20, no. 11:1223-1229.

17. Bray, G.A. "Effect of caloric restriction on energy expenditure of obese patients. Lancet. (1969); 2:397-398.

18. Sims, E., Danforth, E., "Expenditure and Storage of Energy in Man." Journal of Clinic Investigation, (April 1987); 79:1019-1025.

19. Acheson, K., Ravussin, E., "Thermic Effect of Glucose in Man." Journal of Clinical Investigation, (November 1984); 74: 1572-1580.

20. Passmore, R., Swindells, Y.E. "Observations on the respiratory quotients and weight gain of man after eating large quantities of carbohydrates." British Journal of Nutrition. (1963); 17:331-339.

21. Acheson, K.J., Flatt, J.P., Jequier, E. "Glycogen Synthesis Versus Lipogenesis After a 500 Gram Carbohydrate Meal in Man." Metabolism. (December 1982); Vol. 31, no. 12:1234-1240.

22. Thomas, C.D., Peters, J.C., Reed, G.R., et al. "Nutrient balance and energy expenditure during ad libitum feeding of high-fat and high-carbohydrate diets in humans." American Journal of Clinical Nutrition. (1992); 55:934-42.

23. Wood, J.D., Reid, J.T. "The influence of dietary fat on fat metabolism and body fat deposition in meal-feeding and nibbling rats." British Journal of Nutrition. (1975); 34:15-24.

24. Pi-Sunyer, F.X. "Effect of the Composition of the Diet on Energy Intake." Nutrition Reviews. (February 1990); Vol. 48:94-105.

25. Flatt, J.P. "Dietary fat, carbohydrate balance, and weight maintenance: effects of exercise." American Journal of Clinical Nutrition. (1987); 45:296-306.

26. Romieu, I., Willett, W., "Energy Intake and Other Determinants of Relative Weight." American Journal of Clinical Nutrition (1988); 47: 406-412.

Chapter Three

1. Miller, D.S., Mumford, P., Stock, M.J. " Gluttony. Thermogensis in Overeating Man." American Journal of Clinical Nutrition. (November 1967); Vol. 20, no. 11:1223-1229.

2. Himms-Hagen, J. "Cellular Thermogenesis." Annual Review of Physiology. (1976); 38:315-351.

3. Thorne, A., Hallberg, D., and Wahren, J. "Meal-induced thermogenesis in obese patients before and after weight reduction." Clinical Physiology. (1989); 9:481-498.

4. D'Alessio, D.A., Kavle, E.C., Mozzoli, M.A., et al. "Thermic Effect of Food in Lean and Obese Men." Journal of Clinical Investigation. (1988); Vol. 81. 1781-1789.

5. Segal., K.R., Cruz-Noori, A., Santiago, J.C., et al. "Reproducibility of the Thermic Effedt of Food in Lean and Obese Men." Fed. Am. Soc. Exp. Biol. (1991); 5:A554.

6. Acheson, K.J. "Thermic effect of glucose in man: obligatory and facultative thermogenesis." Journal of Clinical Investigation. (1984); 74:1572-1580.

7. Shetty, P.S., Jung, R.T., James, W.P.T., et al. "Postprandial thermogenesis in obesity." Clinical Science. (1981); 60:519-525.

8. Segal, K.R., Lacayanga, I., Dunaif, A., et al. "Impact of body fat mass and percent fat on metabolic rate and thermogenesis in men." American Physiological Society. (1989); 256:E573-E579.

9. Bessard, T., Schultz, Y., Jequier, E. "Energy expenditure and postprandial thermogenesis in obese women before and after weight loss." the American Journal of clinical Nutrition. (November 1983); 38:680-693.

10. Jung, R.T., Shetty, P.S., James, W.P.T., et al. "Reduced thermogenesis in obesity." Nature. (May 24, 1979) ; 279:322-323.

11. Robbins, D.C., Danforth, Jr., E., Horton, E.S., et al. "The Effect of Diet on Thermogenesis in Acquired Lipodystrophy." Metabolism. (September 1979); Vol. 28, no. 9:908-916.

12. Segal, K.R., Gutin, B., Nyman, A.M., et al. "Thermic Effect of Food at Rest, during Exercise, and after Exercise in Lean and Obese Men of Similar Body Weight." Journal of Clinical Investigation. (September 1985); 76:1107-1112.

13. Bessard, T., Schutz, Y., Jequier, E., "Energy Expenditure and Postprandial Thermogenesis in Obese Women Before and After Weightloss." The American Journal of Clinical Nutrition 38. (November 1983); 680-693.

14. Segal, K.R., Albu, J., Chun, A., et al. "Independent Effects of Obesity and Insulin Resistance on Postprandial Thermogenesis in Men." Journal of Clinical Investigation. (March 1992); 89:824-833.

15. Blaza, S., Garrow, J.S. "Thermogenic response to temperature, exercise and food stimuli in lean and obese women, studied by 24 h direct calorimetry." British Journal of Nutrition. (1983); 49:171-180.

16. Golay, A., Schutz, Y., Felber, J.P., et al. "Lack of Thermogenic response to glucose/insulin infusion in diabetic obese subjects."

International Journal of Obesity. (1986); 10:107-116>

17. Crapo, P.A., Reaven, G., Olefsky, J. et al. "Plasma Glucose and Insulin Responses to Orally Administered Simple and Complex Carbohydrates." Diabetes. (September 1976); Vol. 25, 9:741-747.

18. Acheson, K.J., Flatt, J.P., Jequier, E. "Glycogen Synthesis Versus Lipogenesis After a 500 Gram Carbohydrate Meal in Man." Metabolism. (December 1982); Vol. 31, no. 12:1234-1240.

19. Ravussin, E., Acheson, K., "Evidence that insulin resistance is responsible for the decreased thermic effect of glucose in human obesity." Journal of Clinical Investigation. (September 1985); 76: 1268-1273.

20. Reaven, G., Moore, J., "Quantification insulin secretion and in vivo insulin action in non obese and moderately obese individuals with normal glucose tolerance." Diabetes, (July 1983); 32: 600-604.

21. Segal, K., Albu, J., "Independent effects of obesity and insulin resistance on postprandial thermogenesis in men." Journal of Clinical Investigation. (March 1992); 89: 824-833.

22. Sadur, C.N., Yost,T.J., Eckel, R.H. "Fat Feeding Decreases Insulin Responsiveness of Adipose Tissue Lipoprotein Lipase." Metabolism. (November 1984); Vol. 33, no. 11:1043-1047.

23. Bjorntorp, P., Sjostrom,L. "Carbohydrate Storage in Man: Speculations and some Quantative Considerations." Metabolism. (December 1978); Vol. 27, 12,Suppl. 2:1853-1865.

24. Flatt, J.P. "Dietary fat, carbohydrate balance, and weight maintenance: effects of exercise." American Journal of Clinical Nutrition. (1987); 45:296-306.

25. Acheson, K.J., Schutz, Y., Bessard, T., et al. "Nutritional influences on lipogenesis and thermogenesis after a carbohydrate meal." American Journal of Physiology. (January 1984); 246:E62-70.

26. Jenkins, D.J.A., Wolever, T.M.S., Vuksan, V., et al. "Nibbling versus gorging: Metobolic advantages of increased meal frequency." The New England Journal of Medicine. (October 5, 1989); Vol. 321, 14:929-934.

27. Swindells, Yola E., Holmes, S.A., and Robinson, M.F. "The metabolic response of young women to changes in the frequency of meals." British Journal of Nutrition. (1968); 22:667-680.

28. Leveille, G., "Adipose Tissue Metabolism: influence of periodicityof eating and diet composition." Meeting of Experimental Biology. (April 1969).

29. Sheppard, L., Kristal, A.R., Kushi, L.H. "Weight loss in women participating in a randomized trial of low-fat diets." American Journal of clinical Nutrition. (1991); 54:821-828.

Chapter Four

1. Rizek, R.L., Friend, B., Page, L. "Fat in Today's Food Supply-Level of Use and Sources." Journal of the American Oil Chemists' Society. (June 1974); 51:244-250.

2. Danforth, Jr., E. "Diet and obesity." The American Journal of Clinical Nutrition. (May 1985); 41:1132-1145.

3. Sheppard, L., Kristal, A.R., Kushi, L.H. "Weight loss in women participating in a randomized trial of low-fat diets." American Journal of clinical Nutrition. (1991); 54:821-828.

4. Romieu, I., Willett, W.C., Stampfer, M.J., et al. "Energy intake and other determinants of relative weight." American Journal of Clinical Nutrition. (1988); 47:406-12.

5. Horrobin, D.F. "The Regulation of Prostaglandin Biosynthesis by the Manipulation of Essential Fatty Acid Metabolism." Reviews in Pure & Applied Pharmacological Sciences. (1983) Vol. 4, 4:339-383.

6. Crawford, M.A., Hassam, A.G., and Rivers, P.W. "Essential fatty acid requirements in infancy." The American Journal of Clinical Nutrition. (December 1978); 31:2181-2185.

7. Phillipson, B.E., Rothrock, D.W., Connor, W.E. "Reduction of Plasma Lipids, Lipoproteins, and Apoproteins by Dietary Fish Oils in Patients with Hypertriglyderidemia." The New England Journal of Medicine. (May 9, 1985); Vol. 312, 19:1210-1216.

8. Holman, R.T., Lecture, P. "How Essential are Essential Fatty Acids?" Journal of the American Oil Chemists' Society. (October 1978); 55:774A-781A.

9. Beare-Rogers, J.L., Gray, L.M., Hollywood, R. "The linoleic acid and trans fatty acids of margarines." The American Journal of Clinical Nutrition. (September 1979); 32:1805-1809.

10. Coots, R.H. "A comparison of the metabolixm of cis, cis-linoleic, trans, trans-linoleic, and a mixture of cis, trans- and trans, cis-linoleic acids in the rat." Journal of Lipid Research. (1964); 5:473-476.

11. Privett, O.S. "Studies of effects of trans fatty acids in the diet on lipid metabolism in essential fatty acid deficient rats." (July 1977); 30:1009-1017.

12. Vergroesen, A.J. "Dietary fat and cardiovascular disease: possible modes of action of linoleic acid." Proceedings of the Nutrition Society. (1972); 93:175-179.

13. Holman, R.T., Jorgensen, E.A. "Effects of trans Fatty Acid Isoners upon Essential Fatty Acid Deficiency in Rats." Proceedings of the Society for Experimental Biology & Medicine. (1056); 93:175-179.

14. Miljanich, P., Ostwald, R. "Fatty Acids in Newer Brands of Margarine." Journal of the American Dietetic Association. (1970); Vol. 56, no.29:29-30.

15. Thomas, L.H., Jones, P.R., Winter, J.A. et al. "Hydrogenated oils and fats: the presence of chemically-modified fatty acids in human adipose tissue." American Journal of Clinical Nutrition. (May 1981); 34:877-886.

16. Kinsella, J.E., Bruckner, G., Mai., J., et al. "Metabolism of trans fatty acids with emphasis on the effects of trans, trans-octadecadienoate on lipid composition, essential fatty acid, and prostaglandins: an overview." American Journal of Clinical Nutrition. (October 1981); 34:2307-2318.

17. Grundy, S. "Comparison of monounsaturated fatty acids and carbohydrates for lowering plasma cholesterol." The New England Journal of Medicine. (1986); Vol. 314, no. 12:745-748.

18. U.S. Department of Health and Human Services. DHHS (PHS) "Surgeon General's report on nutrition and health." (1988); Publication no. 88: 50211.

19. Thomas, C.D., Peters, J.C., Reed, G.W., et al. "Nutrient balance and energy expenditure during ad libitum feeding of high-fat and high-carbohydrate diets in humans." American Journal of Clinical Nutrition. (1992); 55:934-942.

20. Sims, E., Danforth, E. "Expenditure and Storage of Energy in Man." Journal of Investigation. (April 1987); 79:1019-1025.

21. Flatt, J.P. "Dietary fat, carbohydrate balance, and weight maintenance: effects of exercise." American Journal of Clinical Nutrition. (1987); 45:296-306.

22. Sadur, C., Yost, T. "Fat feeding decreases insulin responsiveness of adipose tissue lipoprotein lipase." Metabolism. (November 1984); 33: no.11:1043-1047.

23. Danforth, Jr., E. "Diet and obesity." The American Journal of Clinical Nutrition. (May 1985); 41:1132-1145.

Chapter Six

1. Flatt, J.P. "Dietary fat, carbohydrate balance, and weight maintenance: effects of exercise." American Journal of Clinical Nutrition. (1987); 45:296-306.

2. Danforth, Jr., E. "Diet and obesity." The American Journal of Clinical Nutrition. (May 1985); 41:1132-1145.

3. Crapo, P.A., Reaven, G., Olefsky, J. et al. "Plasma Glucose and Insulin Responses to Orally Administered Simple and Complex Carbohydrates." Diabetes. (September 1976); Vol. 25, 9:741-747.

4. Swann, D.C., Davidson, P., And Albrink, M.J. "Effect of simple and complex carbohydrates on plasma non-esterified fatty acids, plasma-sugar, and plasma-insulin during oral carbohydrate tolerance tests." Lancet. (1966); I:60-63.

5. Bogardus, C., Lillioja, S., Mott, M., et al. "Relationship between degree of obesity and in vivo insulin action in man." American Journal of Physiology. (1985); 248:E286-E291.

6. Danforth, Jr., E. "The role of thyroid hormones and insulin in the regulation of energy metabolism." The American Journal of Clinical Nutrition. (December 1983); 38:1006-1017

7. Swinburn, B.A., Nyomba, B.L., Saad, M.F., et al. "Insulin Resistance Associated with Lower Rates of Weight Gain in Pima Indians." The Journal of Clinical Investigation. (July 1991); 88:168-173.

8. Ravussin, E., Acheson, K.J., Vernet, O., et al. "Evidence That Insulin Resistance is Responsible for the Decreased Thermic Effect of Glucose in Human Obesity." The Journal of Clinical Investigation. (September 1985); 76:1268-1273.

9. Thorne, A., Hallberg, D., and Wahren, J. "Meal-induced thermogenesis in obese patients before and after weight reduction." Clinical Physiology. (1989); 9:481-498.

10. Reaven, G.M., Moore, J., and Greenfield, M. "Quantification of Insulin Secretion and In Vivo Insulin Action in Nonobese and Moderately Obese Individuals with Normal Glucose Tolerance." Diabetes. (July 1983); 32:600-604.

11. Felig, P. "Hypothesis. Insulin is the mediator of feeding-related thermogenesis: insulin resistance and/or deficiency results in a thermogenic defect which contributes to the pathogenesis of obesity." Clinical Physiology. (1984); 4:267-273.

12. Pi-Sunyer, F.X. "Effect of the Composition of the Diet on Energy Intake." Nutrition Reviews. (February 1990); Vol. 48:94-105.

13. Acheson, K.J., Flatt, J.P., Jequier, E. "Glycogen Synthesis Versus Lipogenesis After a 500 Gram Carbohydrate Meal in Man." Metabolism. (December 1982); Vol. 31, no. 12:1234-1240.

14. Acheson, K.J. "Thermic effect of glucose in man: obligatory and facultative thermogenesis." Journal of Clinical Investigation. (1984); 74:1572-1580.

15. Braitman, L.E. "Obesity and caloric intake: The National Health and Nutrition Examination Survey of 1971-1975." (HANES I). The Journal of Chronic Disease (1985) Vol. 38, no. 9:727-732.

16. Passmore, R., Swindells, Y.E. "Observations on the respiratory quotients and weight gain of man after eating large quantities of carbohydrates." British Journal of Nutrition. (1963); 17:331-339.

17. Bjorntorp, P., Sjostrom,L. "Carbohydrate Storage in Man: Speculations and some Quantative Considerations." Metabolism. (December 1978); Vol. 27, 12,Suppl. 2:1853-1865.

18. Welle, W., Campbell, R.G. "Stimulation of Thermogenesis by Carbohydrate Overfeeding." Journal of Clinical Investigation. (April 1983); 71:916-925.

Chapter Nine

1. Bailey, C. The New Fit or Fat. Houghton Mifflin Company (1991); 167 pp.

2. McArdle, W.D., Katch, F.I., Katch, V.L. "Body Composition Assessment." Exercise Physiology, Lea and Febiger Publishers (1981); Chapter 26:368-391.

3. U.S. Department of Health and Human Services. DHHS (PHS) "Surgeon General's report on nutrition and health." (1988); Publication no. 88: 50211.

4. Roach, M. "The World's Biggest Weight Experts." Health, (March/April); 67-72.

5. Leveille, G. "Adipose Tissue Metabolism: influence of periodicityof eating and diet composition." Meeting of Experimental Biology. (April 1969).

6. Jenkins, D.J.A., Wolever, T.M.S., Vuksan, V., et al. "Nibbling versus gorging: metabolic advantages of increased meal frequency." The New England Journal of Medicine. (October 5, 1987); Vol. 321, 14: 929-934.

7. 4. Braitman, L.E. "Obesity and caloric intake: The National Health and Nutrition Examination Survey of 1971-1975." (HANES I). The Journal of Chronic Disease (1985); Vol. 38, no. 9:727-732.

8. Schlundt, D.G., Hill, J.O. "The role of breakfast in the treatment of obesity: A Randomized Clinical Trial." American Journal of Clinical Nutrition (1992); 55:645-651.

Chapter Eleven

1. Swindells, Y. "The influence of activity and size of meals on caloric response in women." British Journal of Nutrition (1972); 27:65.

2. Flatt, J.P. "Dietary fat, carbohydrate balance, and weight maintenance:effects of exercise." American Journal of Clinical Nutrition (1987); 45:296-306.

3. Blaza, S., Garrow, J.S. "Thermogenic response to temperature, exercise, and food stimuli in lean and obese women, studied by 24h direct calorimetry." British Journal of Nutrition (1983); 49:171.

4. Segal, K., Gutin, B., "Thermic effect of food at rest, during exercise, and after exercise in lean and obese men of similar body weight." Journal of Investigation (September 1985); 76: 1107-1112.

5. Roach, M. "The World's Biggest Weight Experts." Health, (March/April); 67-72.

6. Bailey, C. The New Fit or Fat. Houghton Mifflin Company (1991); 167 pp.

7. Rippe, D. Exercise Exchange Program. Simon & Schuster Trade. (February 1992); 228.

8. Schlundt, D.G., Hill, J.O., "The role of breakfast in the treatment of obesity: A randomized clinical trial." American Journal of Clinical Nutrition (1992); 55: 645-651.